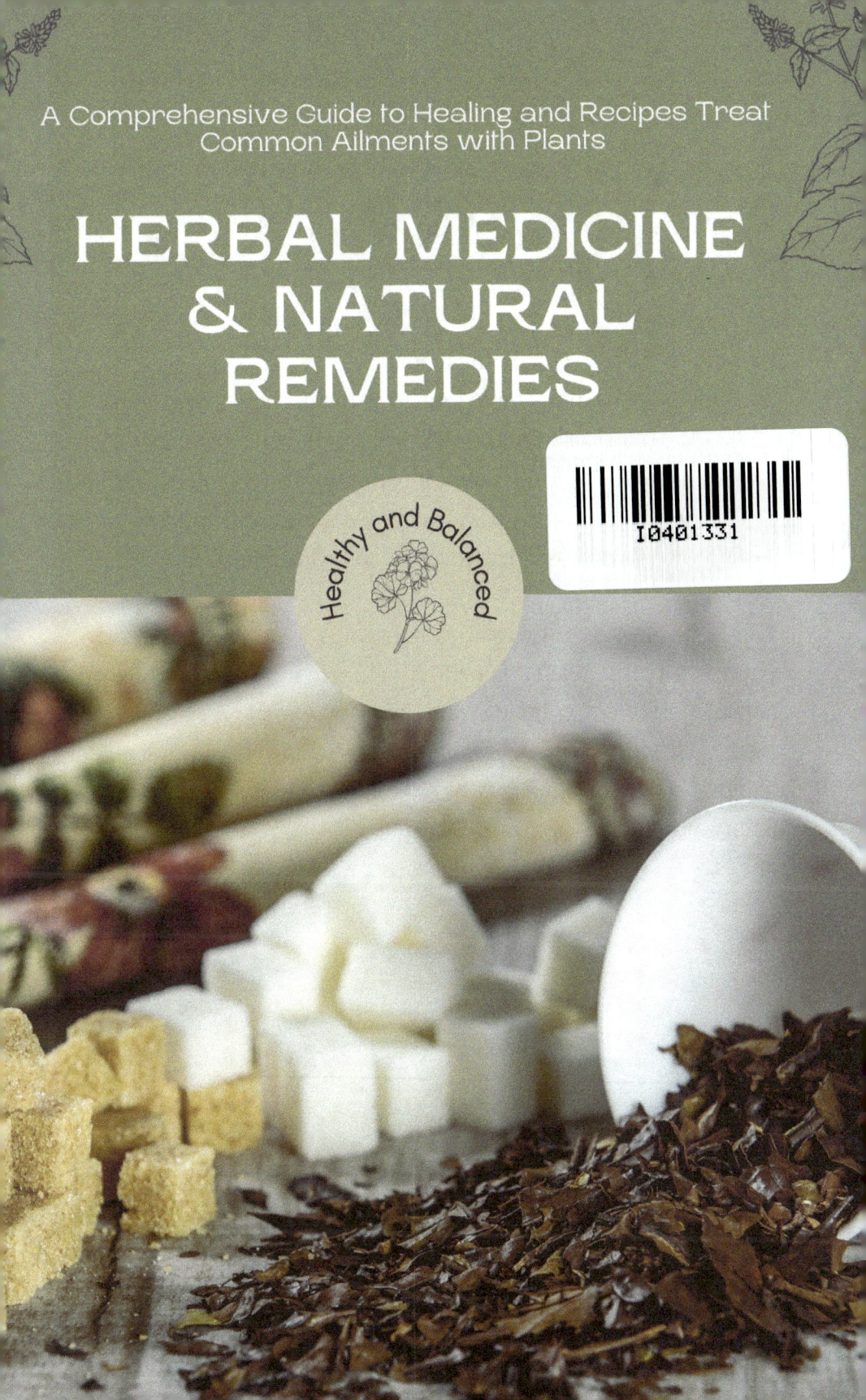

A Comprehensive Guide to Healing and Recipes Treat Common Ailments with Plants

HERBAL MEDICINE & NATURAL REMEDIES

Healthy and Balanced

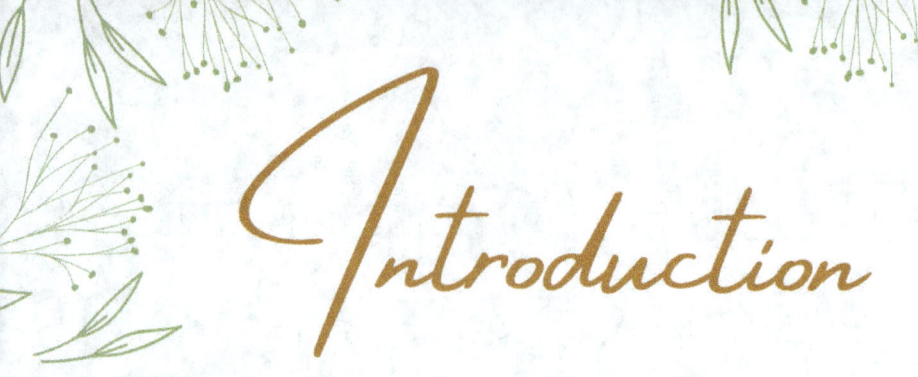

Introduction

Unlocking Nature's Medicine Chest

For millennia, humans have looked to the natural world for healing. Leaves, roots, and flowers have served as our first pharmacies, offering a wealth of remedies for everyday ailments. In this comprehensive guide, "Herbal Medicine & Natural Remedies," we embark on a journey to rediscover this ancient wisdom.

This book is your gateway to harnessing the power of plants for your well-being. We'll delve into the fascinating science behind herbal medicine, exploring how different plants possess unique medicinal properties. Whether you're seeking relief from a nagging cough or aiming to boost your overall health, this guide equips you with the knowledge to choose the right herbs for your needs.

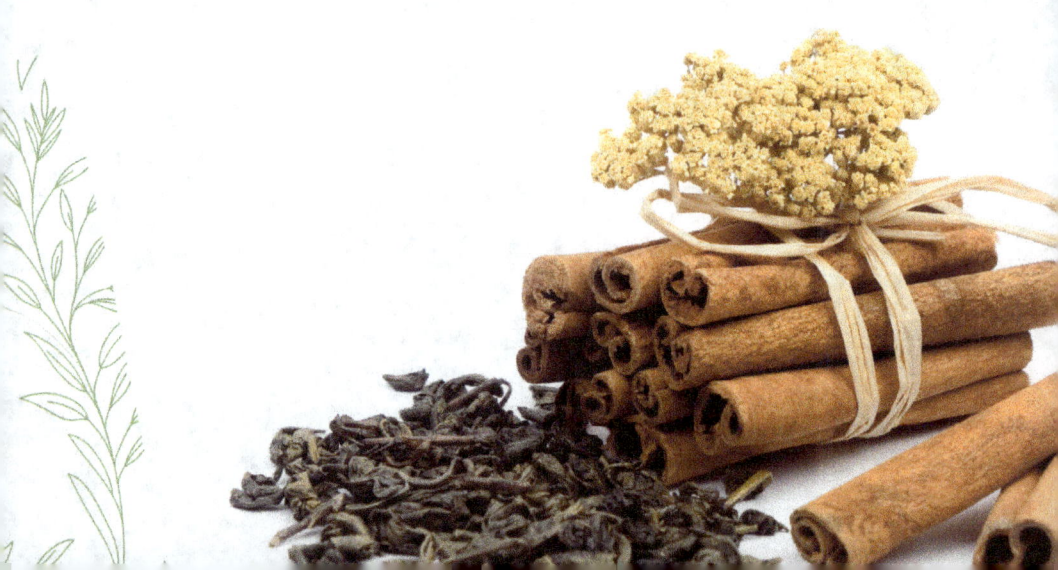

Introduction

Forget harsh chemicals and potentially harmful side effects. We'll explore gentle, natural remedies that work in harmony with your body. You'll learn how to identify common healing plants, prepare safe and effective herbal concoctions, and integrate them seamlessly into your daily routine.

This is more than just a book on herbal remedies; it's an invitation to reconnect with nature's healing power. As you embark on this journey, you'll gain a deeper understanding of your body's natural resilience and discover the profound connection between the plant world and our own well-being.

So, turn the page and let's embark on this exploration of herbal medicine together. With each chapter, you'll unlock a treasure trove of natural remedies waiting to be discovered. Let nature be your guide to a healthier, happier you!

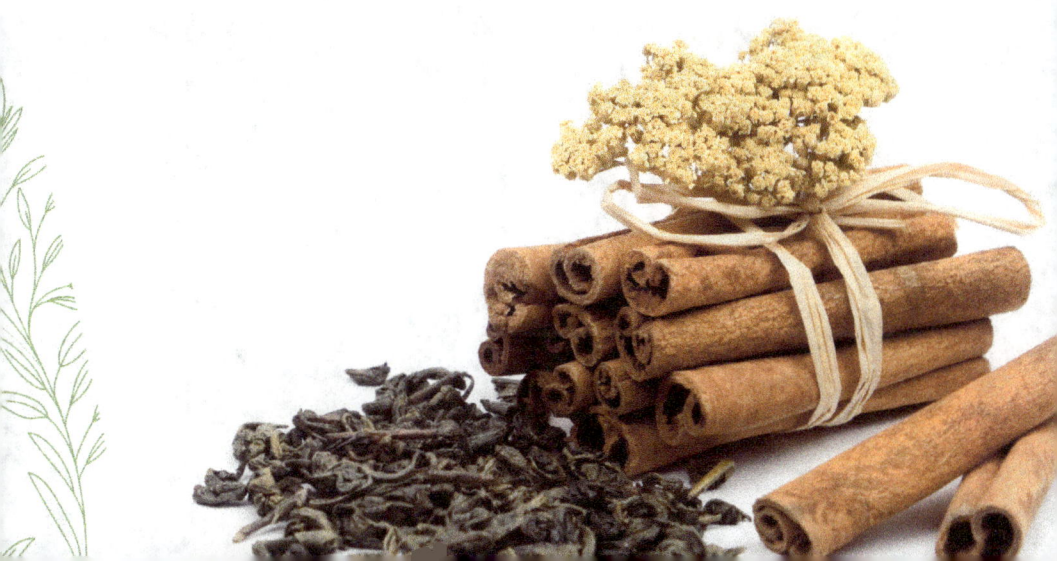

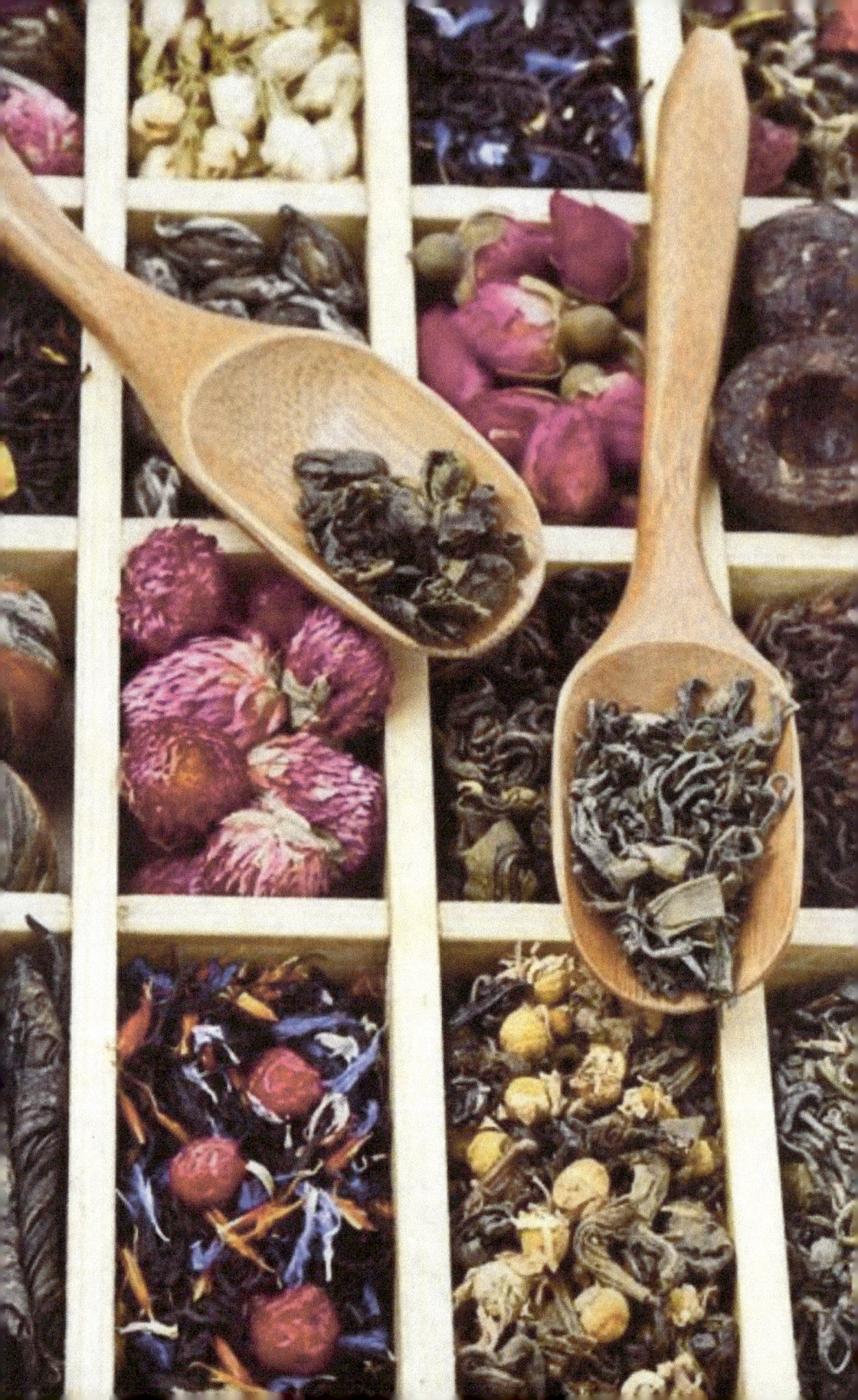

Table of contents

Table of contents

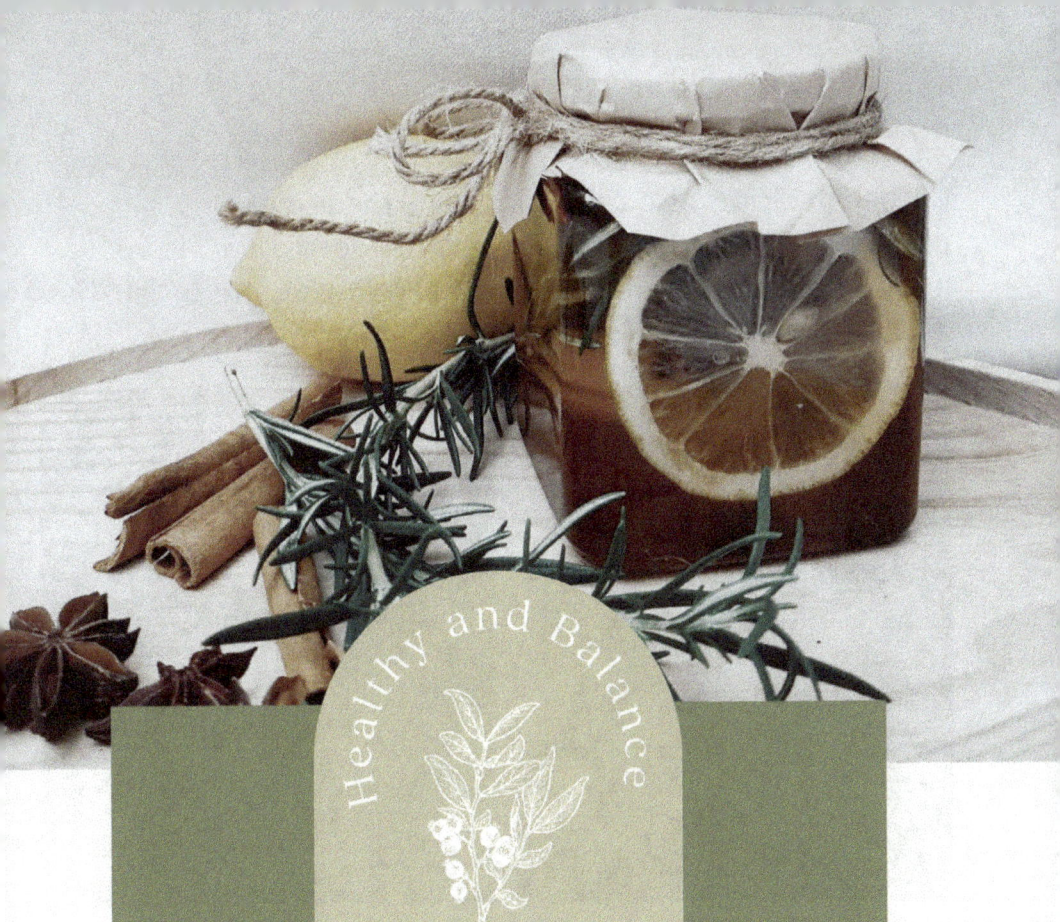

Healthy and Balance

Herbal Medicine

Information you need to know

What is herbal medicine?

Herbal medicine, also called botanical medicine or phytomedicine, refers to using a plant's seeds, berries, roots, leaves, bark, or flowers for medicinal purposes. Herbalism has a long tradition of use outside conventional medicine.

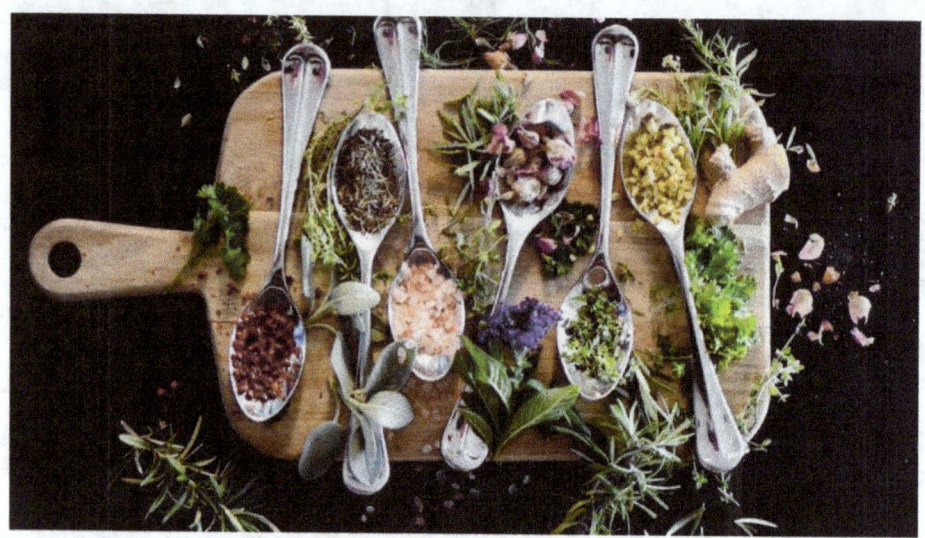

It is becoming more mainstream as improvements in analysis and quality control, along with advances in clinical research, show the value of herbal medicine in treating and preventing disease.

What is the history of herbal medicine?

Plants have been used for medicinal purposes long before recorded history. Ancient Chinese and Egyptian papyrus writings describe medicinal uses for plants as early as 3,000 BC. Indigenous cultures (such as African and Native American) used herbs in their healing rituals, while others developed traditional medical systems (such as Ayurveda and Traditional Chinese Medicine) in which herbal therapies were used.

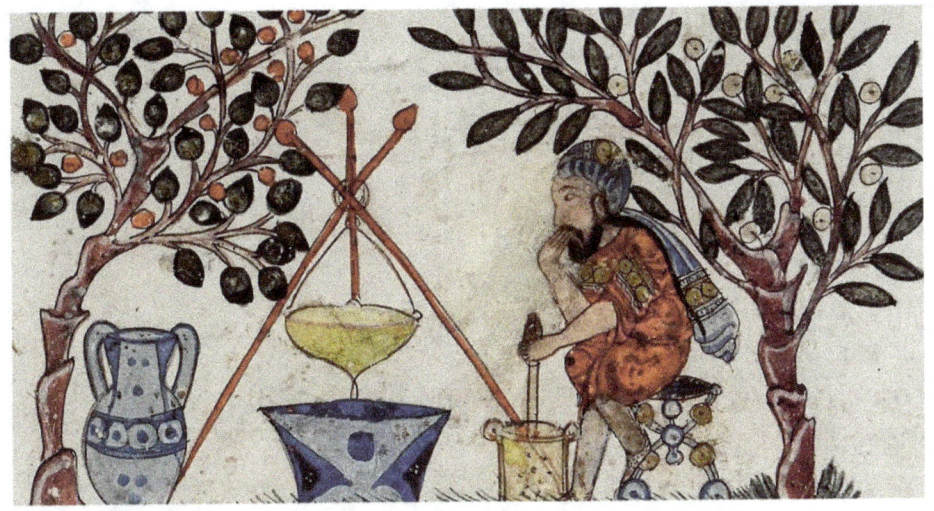

Researchers found that people in different parts of the world tended to use the same or similar plants for the same purposes.

In the early 19th century, when chemical analysis first became available, scientists began to extract and modify the active ingredients from plants. Later, chemists began making their own version of plant compounds and, over time, the use of herbal medicines declined in favor of drugs. Almost one fourth of pharmaceutical drugs are derived from botanicals.

Recently, the World Health Organization estimated that 80% of people worldwide rely on herbal medicines for some part of their primary health care. In Germany, about 600 to 700 plant based medicines are available and are prescribed by some 70% of German physicians. In the past 20 years in the United States, public dissatisfaction with the cost of prescription medications, combined with an interest in returning to natural or organic remedies, has led to an increase in herbal medicine use.

How do herbs work?

In many cases, scientists are not sure what specific ingredient in a particular herb works to treat a condition or illness. Whole herbs contain many ingredients, and they may work together to produce a beneficial effect. Many factors determine how effective an herb will be. For example, the type of environment (climate, bugs, and soil quality) in which a plant grew will affect it, as will how and when it was harvested and processed.

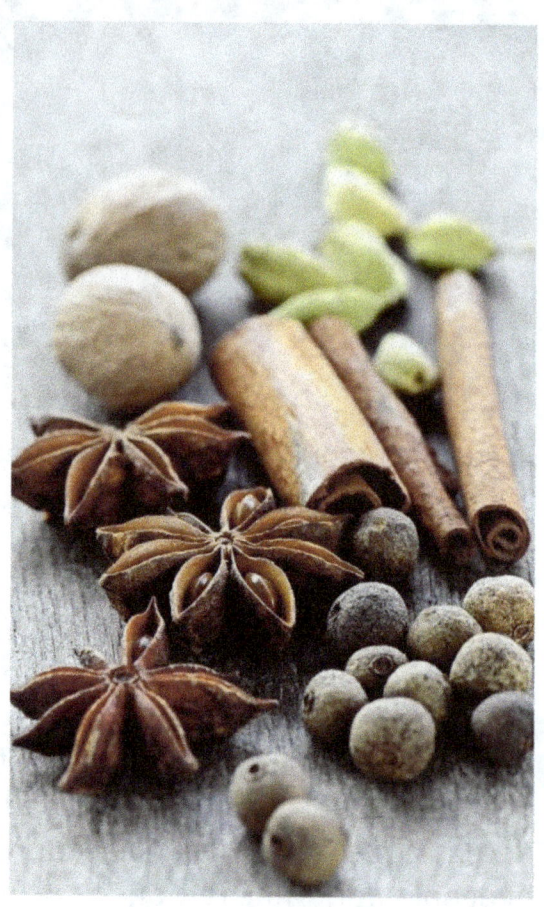

How are herbs used?

The use of herbal supplements has increased dramatically over the past 30 years. Herbal supplements are classified as dietary supplements by the U.S. Dietary Supplement Health and Education Act (DSHEA) of 1994. That means herbal supplements, unlike prescription drugs, can be sold without being tested to prove they are safe and effective. However, herbal supplements must be made according to good manufacturing practices.

The most commonly used herbal supplements in the U.S. include:

- *Echinacea (Echinacea purpurea and related species)*
- *St. John's wort (Hypericum perforatum)*
- *Ginkgo (Ginkgo biloba)*
- *Garlic (Allium sativum)*
- *Saw palmetto (Serenoa repens)*
- *Ginseng (Panax ginseng or Asian ginseng) and Panax quinquefolius or American ginseng)*
- *Goldenseal (Hydrastis canadensis)*
- *Valerian (Valeriana officinalis)*
- *Chamomile (Matricaria recutita)*
- *Feverfew (Tanacetum parthenium)*
- *Ginger (Zingiber officinale)*
- *Evening primrose (Oenothera biennis)*
- *Milk thistle (Silybum marianum)*

Practitioners often use herbs together because the combination is more effective. Health care providers must take many factors into account when recommending herbs, including the species and variety of the plant, the plant's habitat, how it was stored and processed, and whether or not there are contaminants (including heavy metals and pesticides).

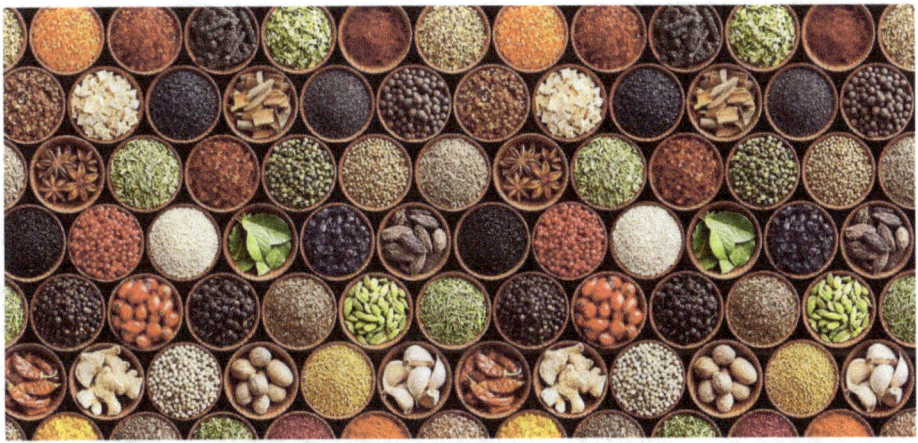

What is herbal medicine good for?

Herbal medicine is used to treat many conditions, such as allergies, asthma, eczema, premenstrual syndrome, rheumatoid arthritis, fibromyalgia, migraine, menopausal symptoms, chronic fatigue, irritable bowel syndrome, and cancer, among others. It is best to take herbal supplements under the guidance of a trained provider. For example, one study found that 90% of people with arthritic use alternative therapies, such as herbal medicine. Since herbal medicines can potentially interact with prescription medications, and may worsen certain medical conditions, be sure to consult with your doctor or pharmacist before taking any herbs. Some common herbs and their uses are discussed below.

- **Ginkgo (Ginkgo biloba)** has been used in traditional medicine to treat circulatory disorders and enhance memory. Although not all studies agree, ginkgo may be especially effective in treating dementia (including Alzheimer disease) and intermittent claudication (poor circulation in the legs). It also shows promise for enhancing memory in older adults. Laboratory studies have shown that ginkgo improves blood circulation by dilating blood vessels and reducing the stickiness of blood platelets. By the same token, this means ginkgo may also increase the effect of some blood-thinning medications, including aspirin. People taking blood-thinning medications should ask their doctor before using ginkgo. People with a history of seizures and people with fertility issues should also use concern; Speak with your physician.

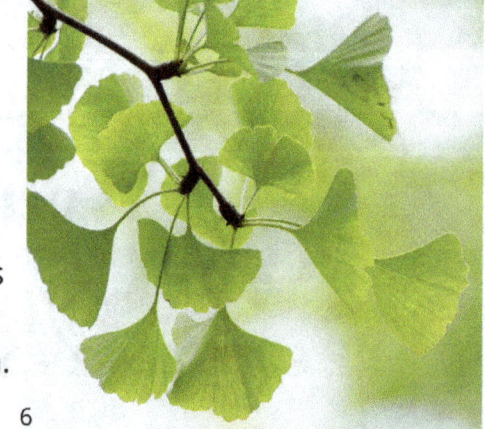

- **Kava kava (Piper methysticum)** is said to elevate mood, enhance wellbeing and contentment, and produce a feeling of relaxation. Several studies show that kava may help treat anxiety, insomnia, and related nervous disorders. However, there is serious concern that kava may cause liver damage. It is not clear whether the kava itself caused liver damage in a few people, or whether it was taking kava in combination with other drugs or herbs. It is also not clear whether kava is dangerous at previously recommended doses, or only at higher doses. Some countries have taken kava off the market. It remains available in the United States, but the Food and Drug Administration (FDA) issued a consumer advisory in March of 2002 regarding the "rare" but potential risk of liver failure associated with kava-containing products.

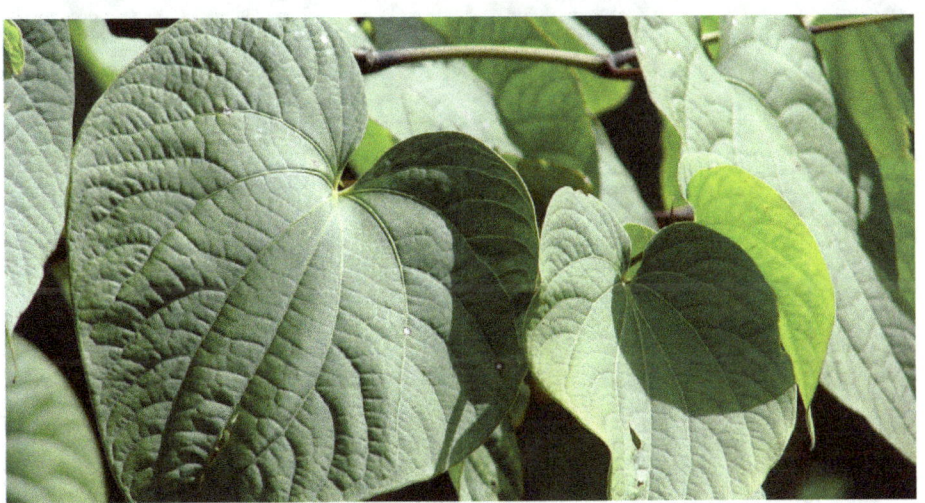

- **Saw palmetto (Serenoa repens)** is used by more than 2 million men in the United States for the treatment of benign prostatic hyperplasia (BPH), a noncancerous enlargement of the prostate gland. Several studies suggest that the herb is effective for treating symptoms, .

including frequent urination, having trouble starting or maintaining urination, and needing to urinate during the night. But not all studies agree. At least one well-conducted study found that saw palmetto was no better than placebo in relieving the signs and symptoms of BPH

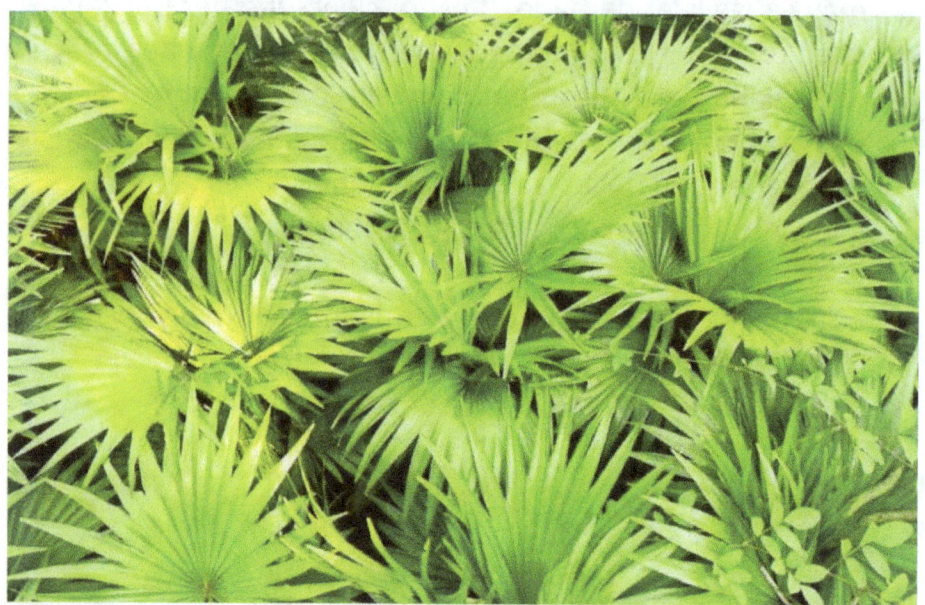

- **St. John's wort (Hypericum perforatum)** is well known for its antidepressant effects. In general, most studies have shown that St. John's wort may be an effective treatment for mild-to-moderate depression, and has fewer side effects than most other prescription antidepressants. But the herb interacts with a wide variety of medications, including birth control pills, and can potentially cause unwanted side effects, so it is important to take it only under the guidance of a health care provider.

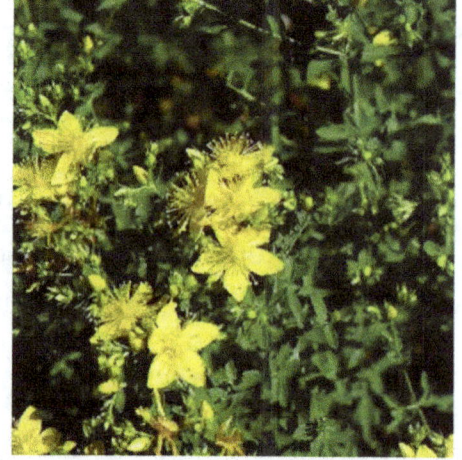

- **Valerian (Valeriana officinalis)** is a popular alternative to commonly prescribed medications for sleep problems because it is considered to be both safe and gentle. Some studies bear this out, although not all have found valerian to be effective. Unlike many prescription sleeping pills, valerian may have fewer side effects, such as morning drowsiness. However, Valerian does interact with some medications, particularly psychiatric medications, so you should speak to your doctor to see if Valerian is right for you.

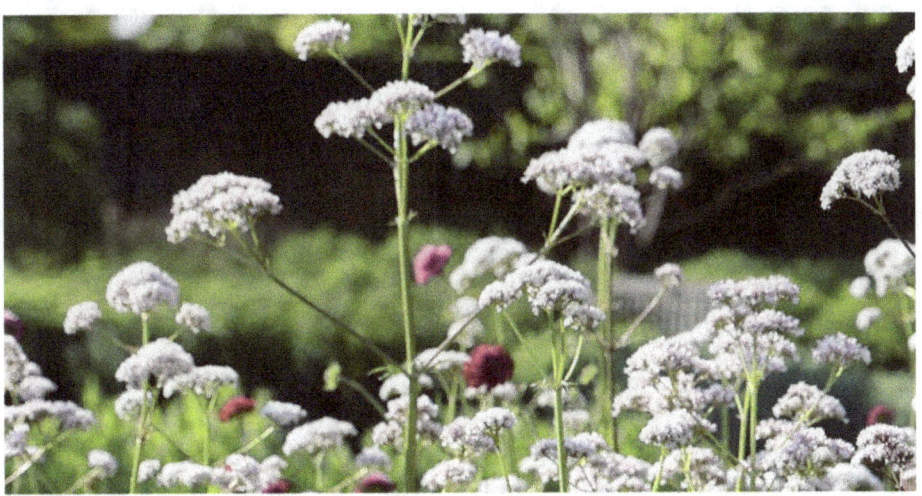

- **Echinacea preparations (from Echinacea purpurea and other Echinacea species)** may improve the body's natural immunity. Echinacea is one of the most commonly used herbal products, but studies are mixed as to whether it can help prevent or treat colds. A review of 14 clinical studies

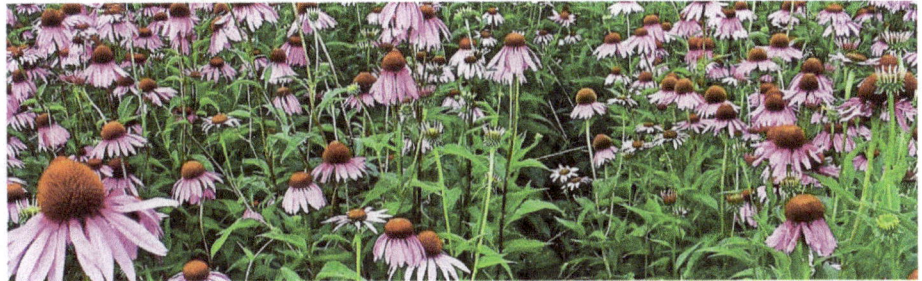

examining the effect of echinacea on the incidence and duration of the common cold found that echinacea supplements decreased the odds of getting a cold by 58%. It also shortened the duration of a cold by 1.4 days. Echinacea can interact with certain medications and may not be right for people with certain conditions, for example people with autoimmune disorders or certain allergies. Speak with your physician.

Is there anything I should watch out for?

Used correctly, herbs can help treat a variety of conditions, and in some cases, may have fewer side effects than some conventional medications. Never assume that because herbs are "natural," they are safe. Some herbs may be inappropriate for people with certain medical conditions. Because they are unregulated, herbal products are often mislabeled and may contain additives and contaminants that are not listed on the label. Some herbs may cause allergic reactions or interact with conventional drugs, and some are toxic if used improperly or at high doses. Taking herbs on your own increases your risk, so it is important to consult with your doctor or pharmacist before taking herbal medicines. Some examples of adverse reactions from certain popular herbs are described below.

- St. John's wort can cause your skin to be more sensitive to the sun's ultraviolet rays, and may cause an allergic reaction, stomach upset, fatigue, and restlessness. Clinical studies have found that St. John's wort also interferes with the effectiveness of many drugs, including the blood thinner warfarin (Couamdin), protease inhibitors for HIV, birth control pills, certain asthma drugs, and many other medications. In addition, St. John's wort should not be taken with prescribed antidepressant medication. The FDA has issued a public health advisory concerning many of these interactions.

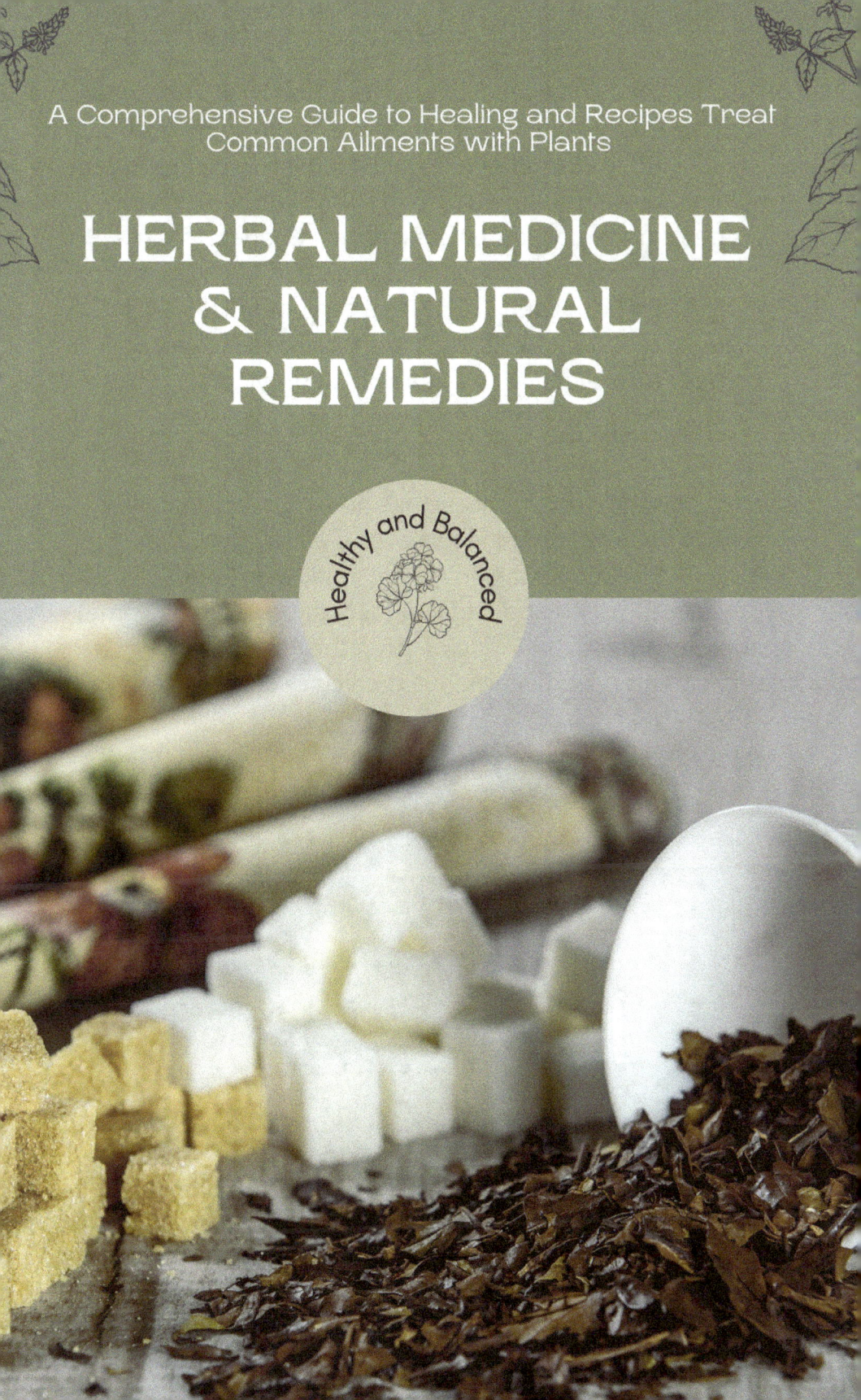

A Comprehensive Guide to Healing and Recipes Treat
Common Ailments with Plants

HERBAL MEDICINE
& NATURAL
REMEDIES

Healthy and Balanced

- St. John's wort (Hypericum perforatum) is well known for its antidepressant effects. In general, most studies have shown that St. John's wort may be an effective treatment for mild-to-moderate depression, and has fewer side effects than most other prescription antidepressants. But the herb interacts with a wide variety of medications, including birth control pills, and can potentially cause unwanted side effects, so it is important to take it only under the guidance of a health care provider.

Who is using herbal medicine?

Nearly one-third of Americans use herbs. Unfortunately, a study in the New England Journal of Medicine found that nearly 70% of people taking herbal medicines (most of whom were well educated and had a higher-than-average income) were reluctant tell their doctors that they used complementary and alternative medicine (CAM).

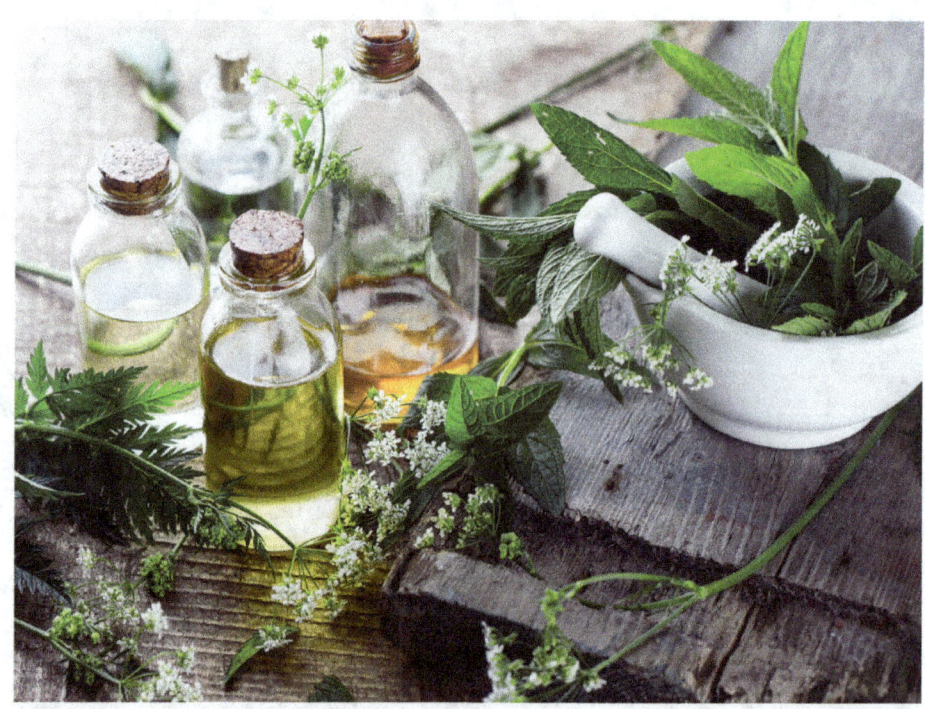

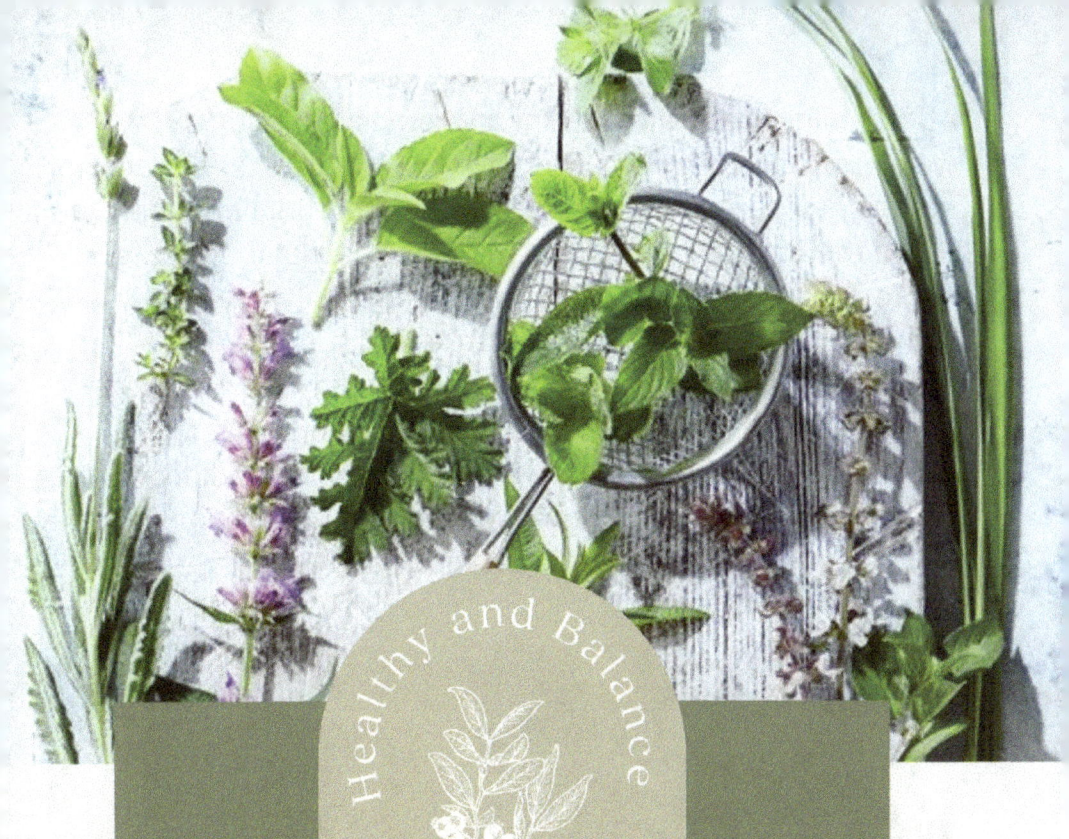

DIY Herbal Recipes You Can Make

Affordability is a real issue when it comes to health and wellness. Many of us are living on tight budgets, and that's not getting any better with the current skyrocketing inflation. One of the things that I love about herbalism is that it empowers me to make better choices for my health and wellbeing without blowing my budget. It's true that some herbal formulations require ingredients that are beyond what I can purchase, but there are many effective options that fall comfortably in the affordable zone, so I've never felt like I missed out because I couldn't buy those pricier options. From wellness recipes to topical applications and culinary treats, these excellent. Enjoy!

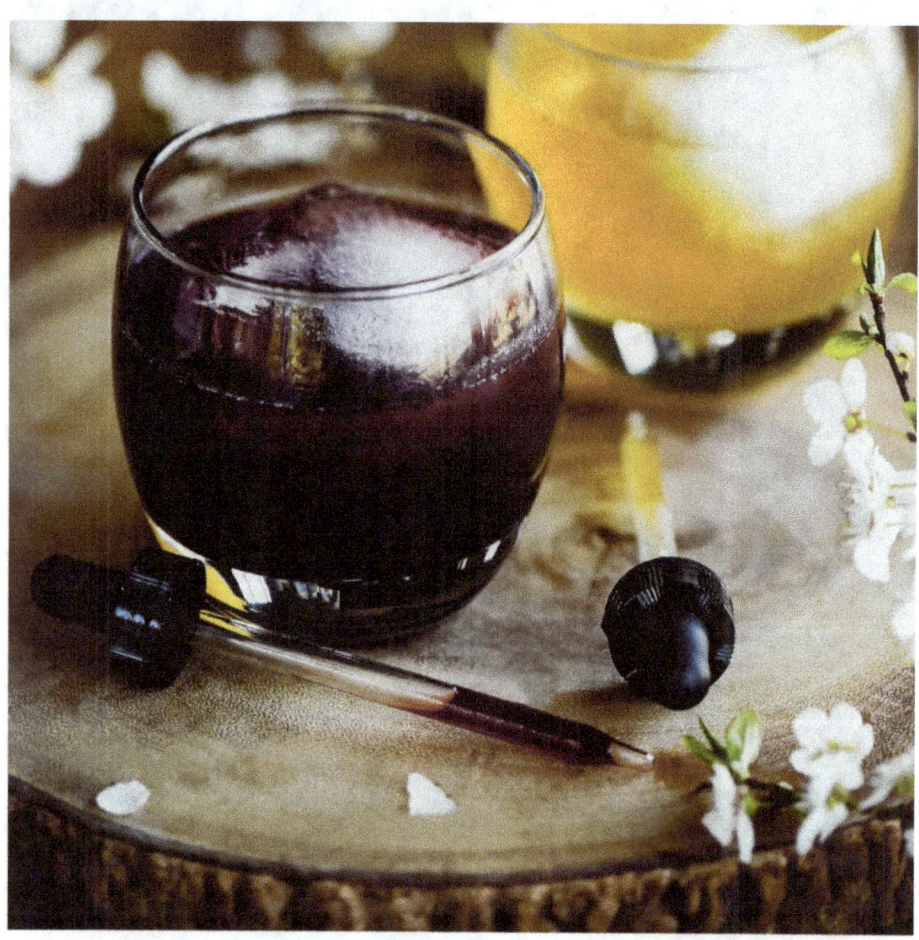

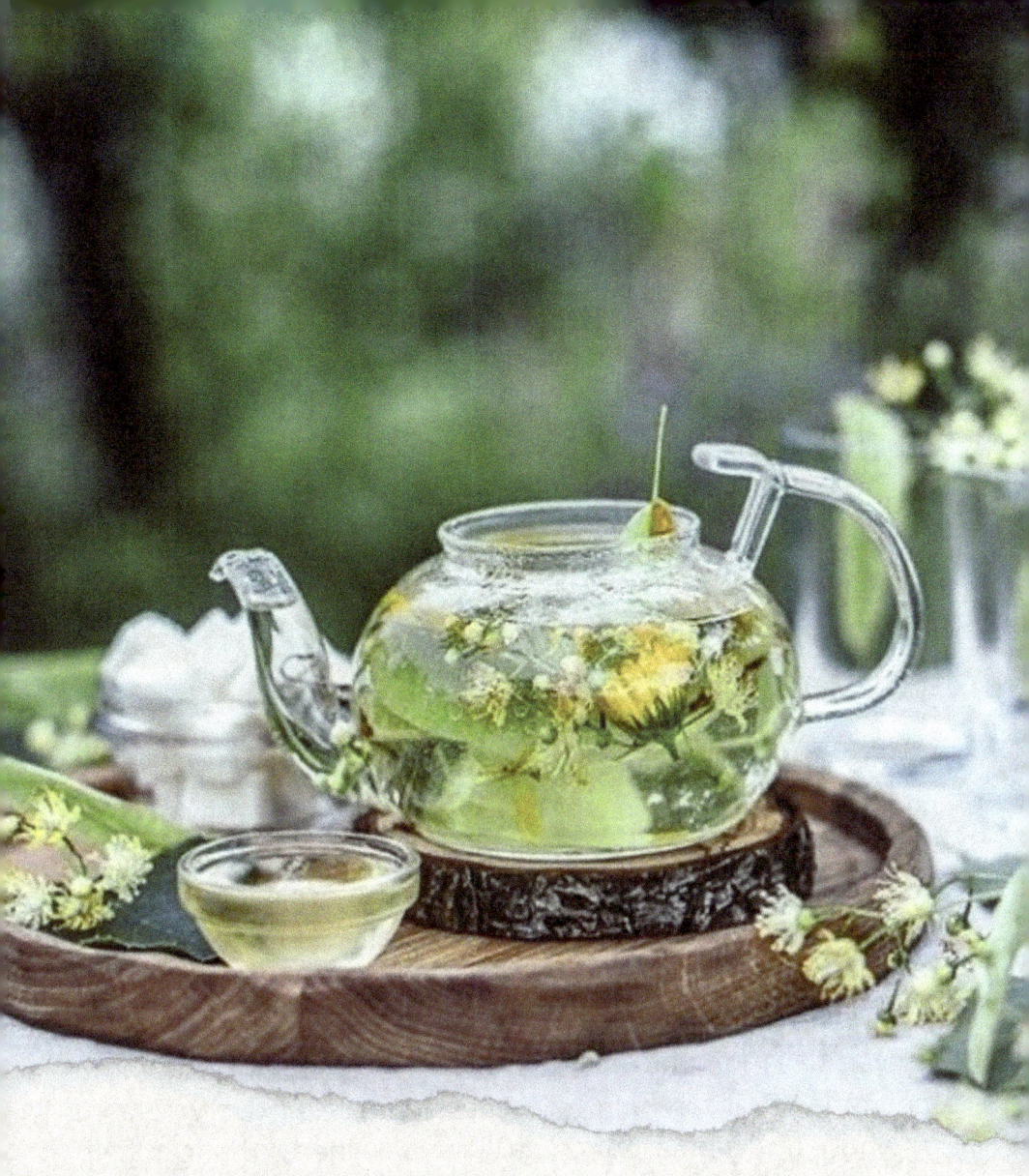

3 TEA RECIPES TO INCREASE MINDFULNESS AND STRESS LESS

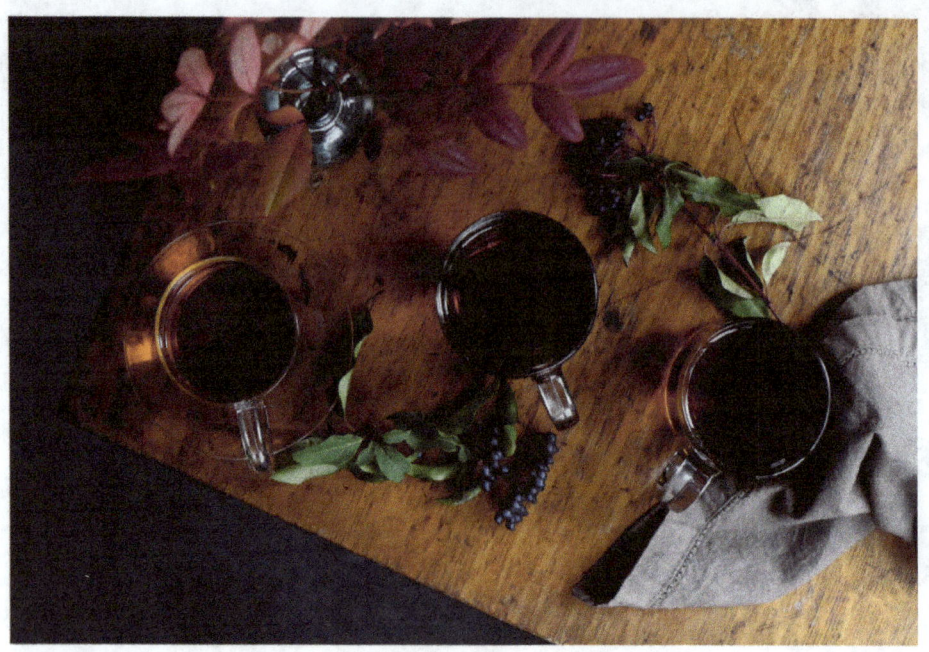

Everyone deals with stress. In fact, stress is said to be the top health problem in America. To keep ourselves healthy and happy, some are turning to the practice of mindfulness. I'm one of those people that thought mindfulness might be worth a try. Since I'm also a fan of tea, I naturally wondered if tea recipes could help with relaxation.

What is mindfulness? Simply put, it's when you're fully present to everyday moments and sensations. It's a kind of ongoing meditation that can help you be less reactive or overwhelmed by what's going on around you. There are herbs that can help do the same thing, so it certainly made sense to me that tea could help increase mindfulness.

The recipes I've selected here extend my sense of calm throughout the day: morning, afternoon, and evening. Feel free to play with the ratios to find the best cup of tea for your needs. Also, when preparing tea throughout the day, I try to remember to slow down and appreciate the aroma and the warmth of the mug as the tea steeps. Then, the best part is savoring that first sip. Preparing and drinking tea can be a mindfulness practice in and of itself.

Lately I've been enjoying specific herbal tea blends to help with mindfulness and stress reduction. They include herbs that have both nervine and adaptogenic properties. These are herbs like skullcap, schisandra berries, holy basil, lemon balm, and chamomile.

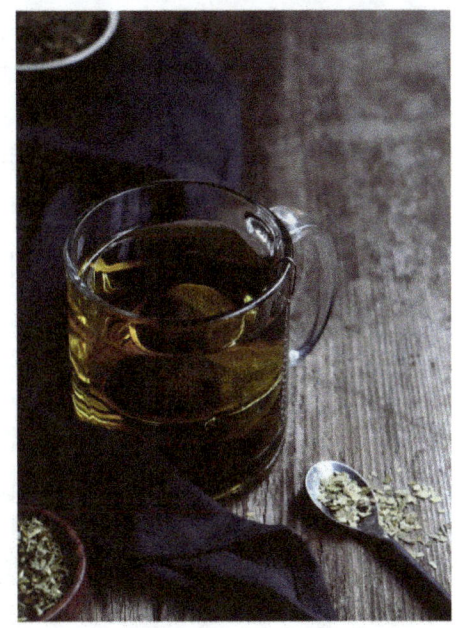

Good Morning Tea

Coffee is great, but for me it's rather overpowering. I've found this tea blend to provide a mellower alternative that keeps me attentive to the task at hand without the jitters.

Ingredients

- 1 tsp. organic skullcap leaf
- 1 tsp. organic peppermint leaf
- 1 Tbsp. organic Yerba mate

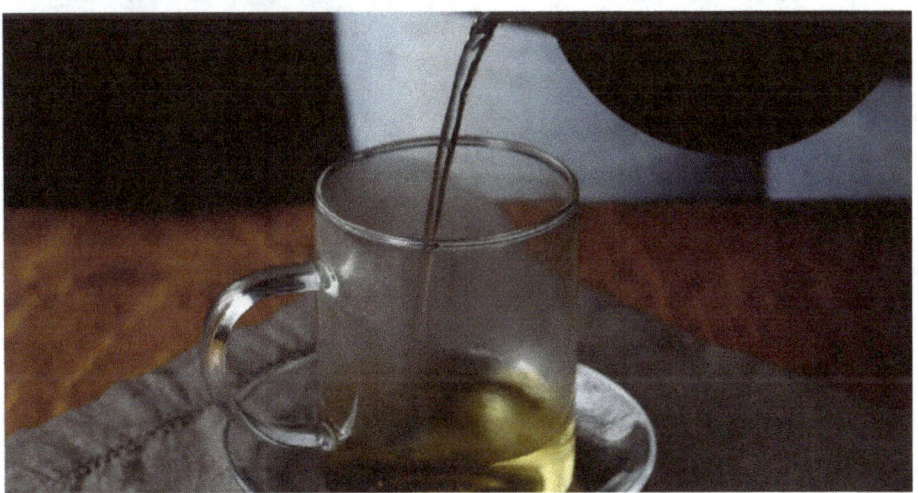

Skullcap not only has a cool name, its nutrients support the nervous system and thus helps ease away everyday stress. Peppermint has a refreshing taste that eases my digestion and gently amplifies my mental focus.

Yerba Mate is packed with vitamins, minerals, amino acids, antioxidants, and caffeine for a stimulating boost that is mellower than coffee.

Midday Mellow Tea

Need an afternoon reminder to mellow out? This sweet tea combines lemon balm and holy basil with a splash of berry. Personally, I enjoy sweetening up this tea with some stevia leaf to really bring out the fruity flavors.

Ingredients

- 1 tsp. organic lemon balm
- 1 Tbsp. organic holy basil
- 1 tsp. organic Schisandra berries
- 1 tsp. organic stevia leaf

Lemon balm can elevate mood and reduce restlessness.

Holy Basil is an important adaptogenic herb in Ayurvedic healing traditions, where it is used to help the mind adapt to incoming stressors.

Schisandra berries are said to calm the heart and quiet the spirit.

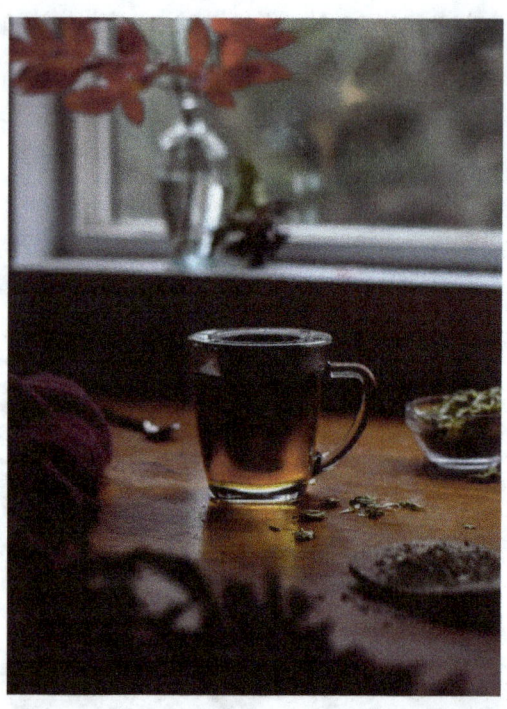

Sunset Tea

Ready to wind down? To prepare my mind for sleep, I find this tea a delicious way to peacefully slow down and drift into dreamland. Start sipping on this relaxing blend one hour before bed.

Ingredients
- 1 tsp. organic hops flowers
- 1 tsp organic mugwort herb
- 1 tsp. organic catnip leaf

Hops have a wonderful way of inducing a sense of inner-peace and calm before bedtime.

Mugwort is a powerful sleepy-time tonic which can assist in manifesting pleasant dreams.

Catnip has calming properties which also can help ease digestion during the night.

For me, incorporating all of these herbs into my daily tea rituals has enhanced my everyday mindfulness. Wherever you are on your journey to greater health and wellbeing, herbal tea preparation and consumption could prove an effective stress reduction strategy for you, as well.

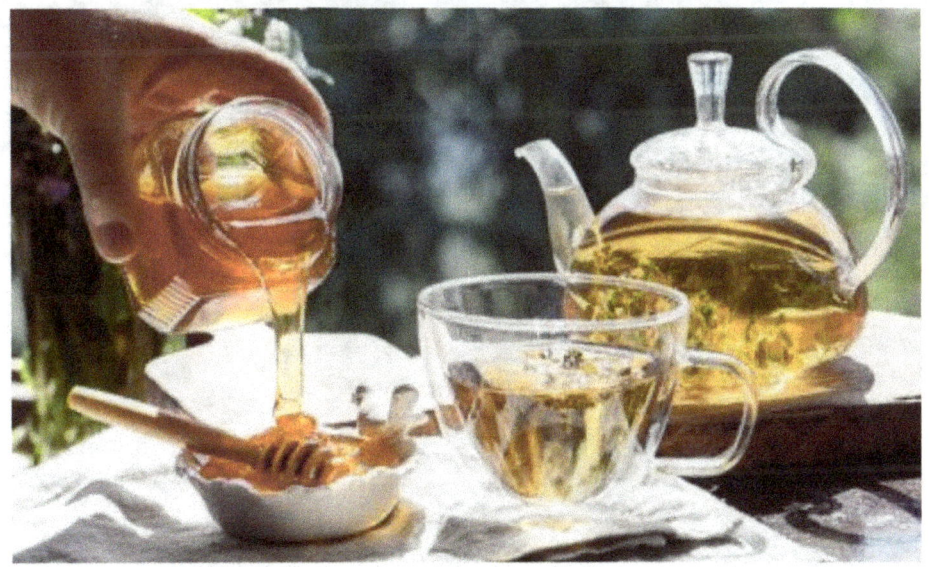

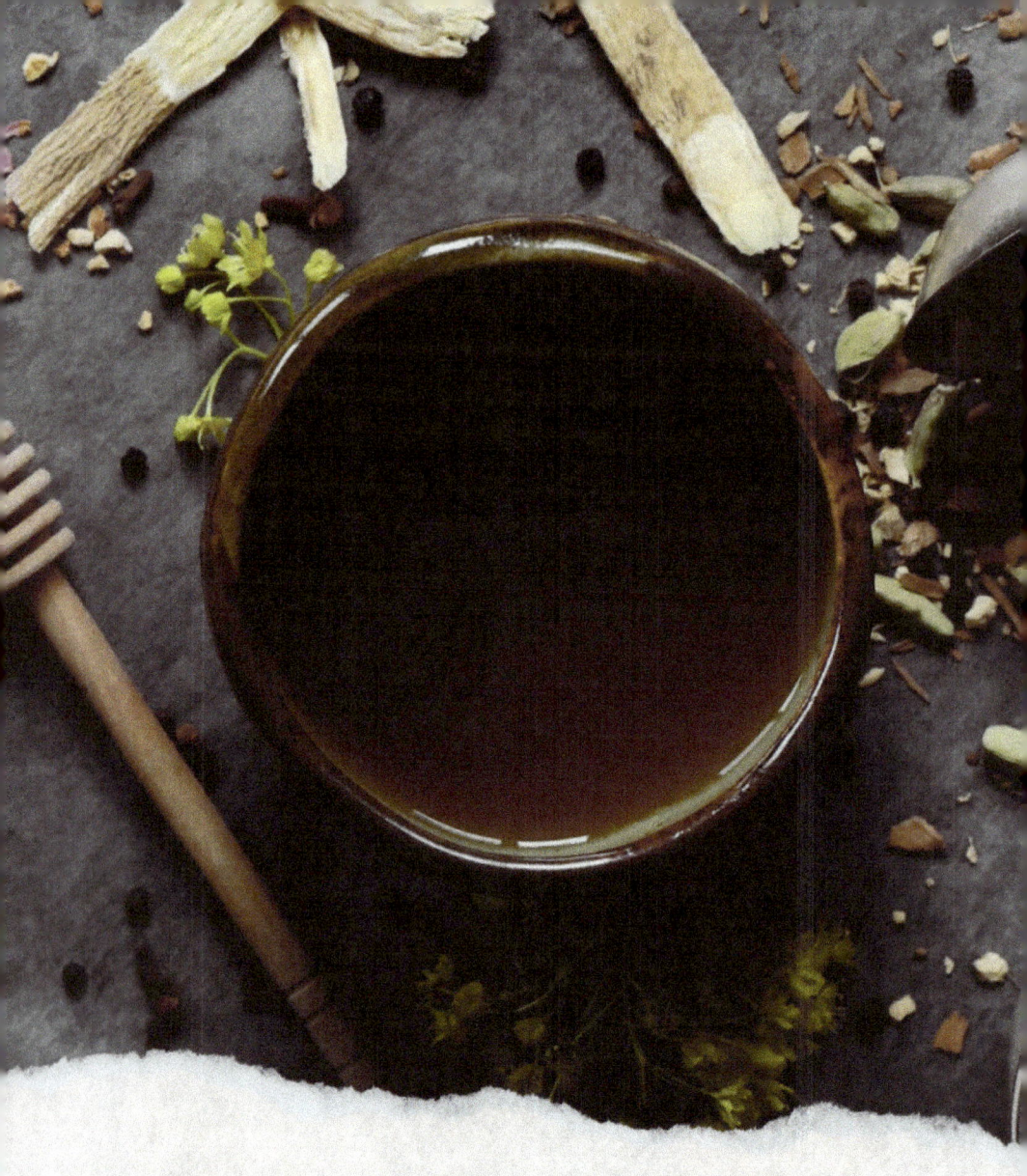

ADAPTOGENIC CHAI TEA RECIPE WITH ASTRAGALUS

If you've ever checked the ingredients list on your favorite chai blend, you may have found yourself dizzied by the long list of herbs and spices involved. While such an assortment might take some work to assemble, this variety also makes chai spice recipes a delicious way to enjoy a whole host of beneficial botanicals in a single cup. And one of our favorite additions, from both a flavor and wellness perspective, is sweet and adaptogenic astragulus root.

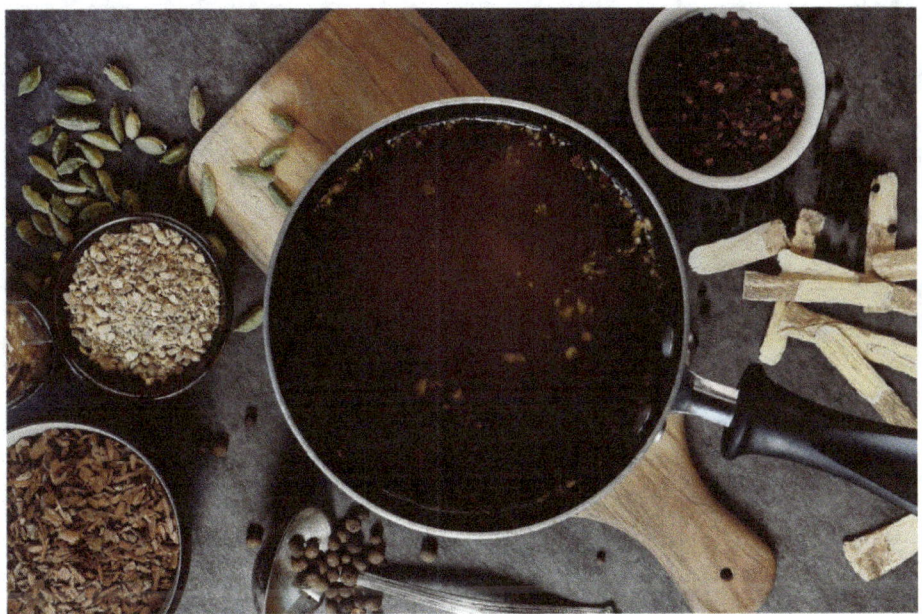

There are countless variations of chai to enjoy (we offer several in our online shop!), but all contain some balance of warming and sweet flavors. Some of the essential "pumpkin spice" elements, such as cinnamon, ginger root, cloves, and cardamom, appear in most recipes (which is one reason chai is so popular during autumn and winter). This classic base pairs well with a surprising range of flavors, making it fun and easy to create tea custom blends to complement your personal tastes and wellness goals—and if one of those goals is immune system support, astragalus root is an excellent addition. *

Astragalus has been found to support immune health and help the body adapt to stress in a healthy way. In fact, it is considered the "king" ingredient in the Traditional Chinese Medicine formula known as Jade Windscreen, a blend taken for protection against spring health threats.

Astragalus Chai Recipe for Immune Support

Makes 6 cups.

Ingredients

- 2 Tbsp. astragalus root or 10-15 small organic astragalus root slices
- 10 slices of organic Chinese licorice root
- 2 Tbsp. of organic ginger root
- 2 Tbsp. organic dried orange peel
- 1 Tbsp. of organic sweet cinnamon chips
- 1 tsp. of organic white peppercorns
- 1-2 organic cardamom pods
- 3-5 organic whole allspice berries
- 3-5 whole organic cloves
- 1 and 1/2 quarts of water

Directions

1. Combine all the ingredients in a saucepan.
2. Bring to a boil.
3. Simmer for one hour.
4. Strain.
5. Add milk and raw, local honey if desired.

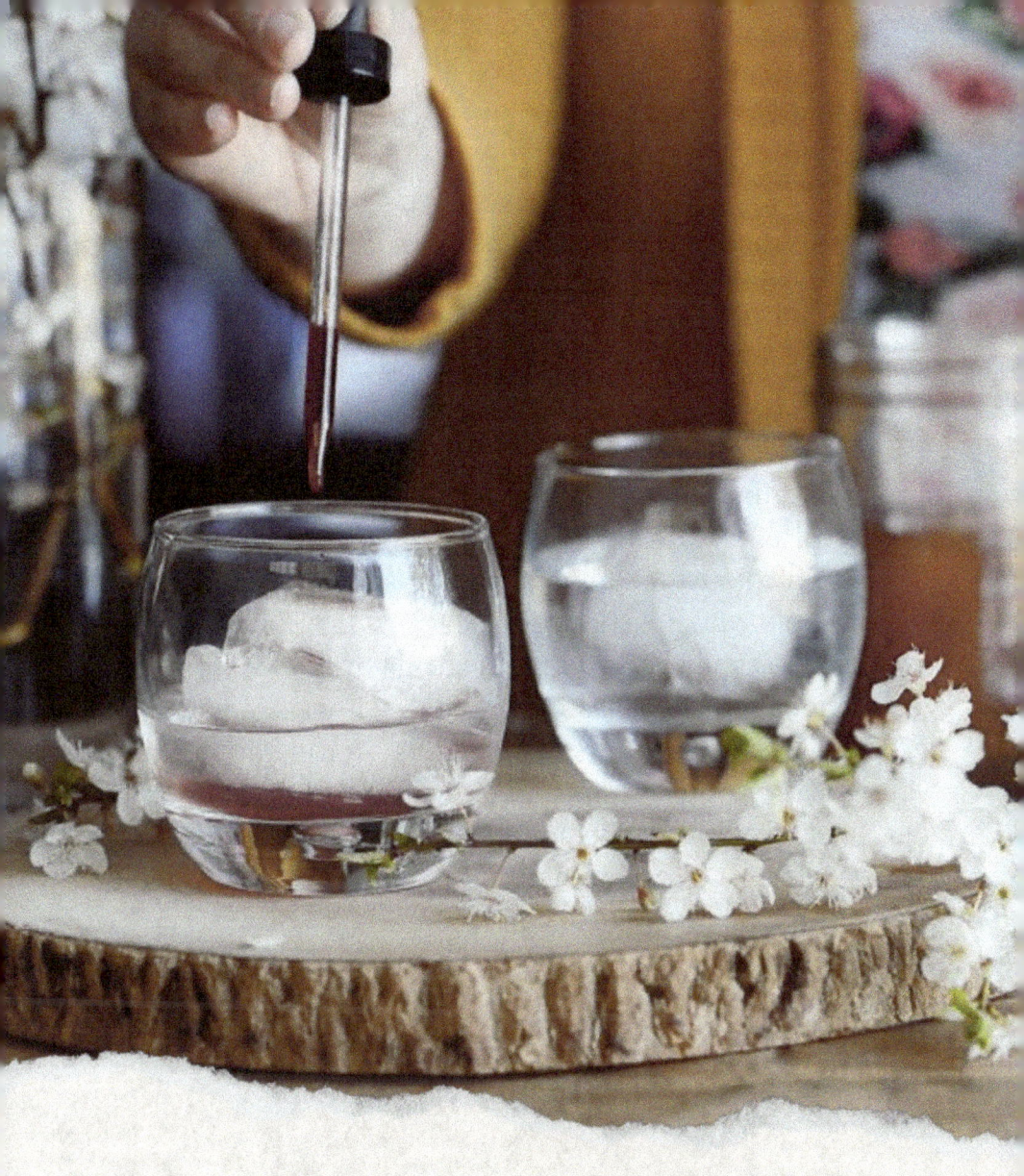

HERBAL OXYMEL
RECIPES & BENEFITS

In 400 B.C.E., in his On Regimen in Acute Diseases, Hippocrates wrote, "You will find the drink, called oxymel, often very useful...for it promotes expectoration and freedom of breathing." It's too bad I didn't have that definition the first time I saw the word "oxymel," because I came across the term right about the same time that I was reading the Harry Potter series to my daughter. This might explain why an oxymel sounds to me like something one would whip up in potions class.

The first definition for oxymel that I found didn't help dispel that magical picture: an oxymel is a type of "herbal elixir"...which puts me in mind of Julie Andrews announcing that "people who get their feet wet must learn to take their medicine" as she spoons out a magical, multi-flavored syrup (rum punch for me, please). While an oxymel is indeed an herbal elixir, not all elixirs are oxymels—for instance, sipping vinegars like fruity shrubs and gingery switchels are delicious herbal elixirs, but they're not necessarily sweetened with honey, which is a requirement for oxymels. I finally landed on

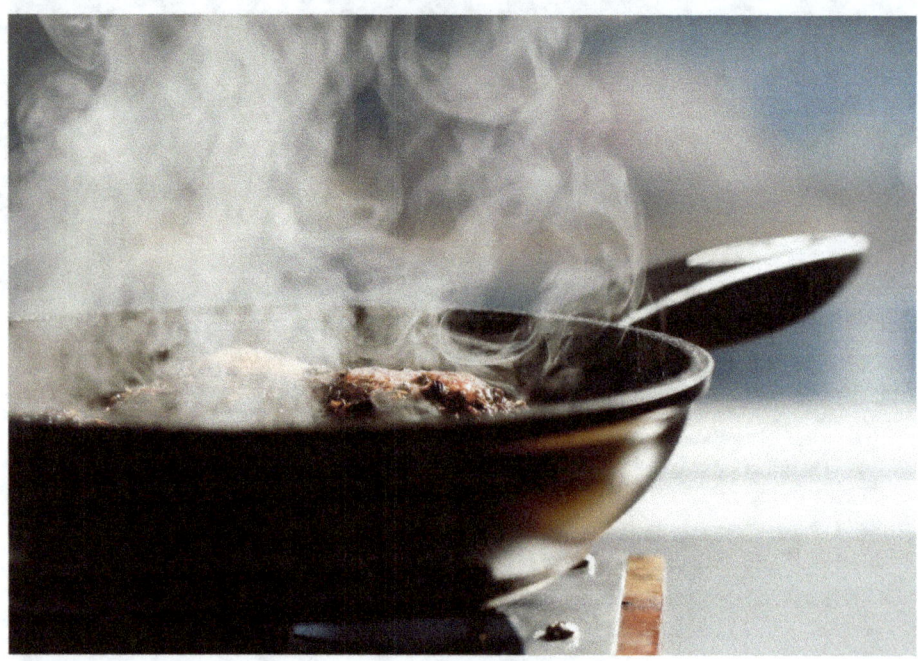

an example of an oxymel that gave me better clarity: when made with honey, fire cider—popularized by esteemed folk herbalist Rosemary Gladstar, and recently the subject of a federal court case over the right to keep traditional remedies trademark-free—is a renowned and beloved immune-supportive oxymel.

Basic Herbal Oxymel Recipe

Ingredients
- Organic dried herbs of choice (see below for some of our favorites)
- 1 part organic, raw apple cider vinegar
- 1 part raw, local honey

Directions
- Depending on what herbs you're using, there are several ways to prepare an oxymel. Here are three great options.

OXYMEL METHOD 1: STIR, SHAKE, SIT

Works well for infusing a variety of dried herbs.
- Fill a pint jar 1/4 full of your choice of herbs.
- Cover with equal parts apple cider vinegar and honey to fill jar.
- Stir to incorporate.
- Wipe any liquid off the rim and top with a tight-fitting plastic lid. Alternatively, place a piece of parchment paper under a metal canning lid and ring to keep the vinegar from touching the metal.
- Shake jar until thoroughly mixed.
- Store jar in a cool, dark place to extract for two weeks. Shake jar at least twice a week to assist in extraction.
- Strain out herbs through a fine mesh strainer, pressing down on the herbs to release as much liquid as possible, retaining liquid and setting herbs aside to compost.
- Pour strained oxymel into glass storage jars or bottles.

- Label and date.
- Store in cool, dark place until ready to use. When stored properly, shelf life is approximately 6 months.

OXYMEL METHOD 2: VINEGAR DECOCTION

Great for non-delicate herbs and hearty roots, or if you're in a pinch and need an oxymel quickly. This heat-based method is too harsh for most highly aromatic or floral herbs.

- Place the dried herbs and twice as much vinegar as you ultimately want into a pot.
- Bring to a boil. (*Be careful! Apple cider vinegar steam can be very intense—don't put your face and eyes over the pot or inhale too much vinegar steam!)
- Reduce heat and allow to simmer gently until the liquid is reduced by about half, usually 30 to 40 minutes.
- Remove from heat and set aside to cool to room temperature.
- Strain out herbs through a fine mesh strainer, pressing down on the herbs to release as much liquid as possible, retaining liquid and setting herbs aside to compost.
- Mix the herbal, decocted vinegar with equal parts honey until thoroughly blended.
- Pour oxymel into glass storage jars or bottles.
- Label and date.
- Store in cool, dark place until ready to use. When stored properly, shelf life is approximately 6 months.

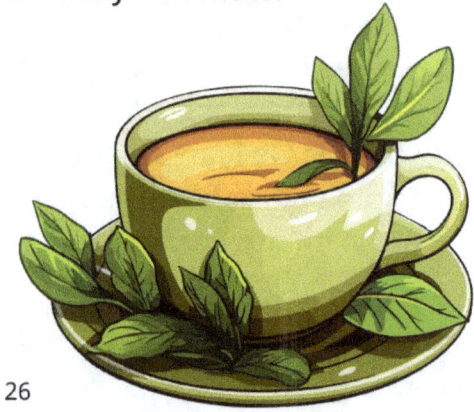

OXYMEL METHOD 3: SEPARATELY INFUSE HONEY AND APPLE CIDER VINEGAR

A nice option for especially delicate herbs.

This is an easy way to make an oxymel if you already have infused honey and/or infused apple cider vinegar in your kitchen pantry or home apothecary.

- Combine equal parts herb-infused honey and herb-infused vinegar in a glass storage jar or bottle.
- Label and date.
- Store in cool, dark place until ready to use. When stored properly, shelf life is approximately 6 months.

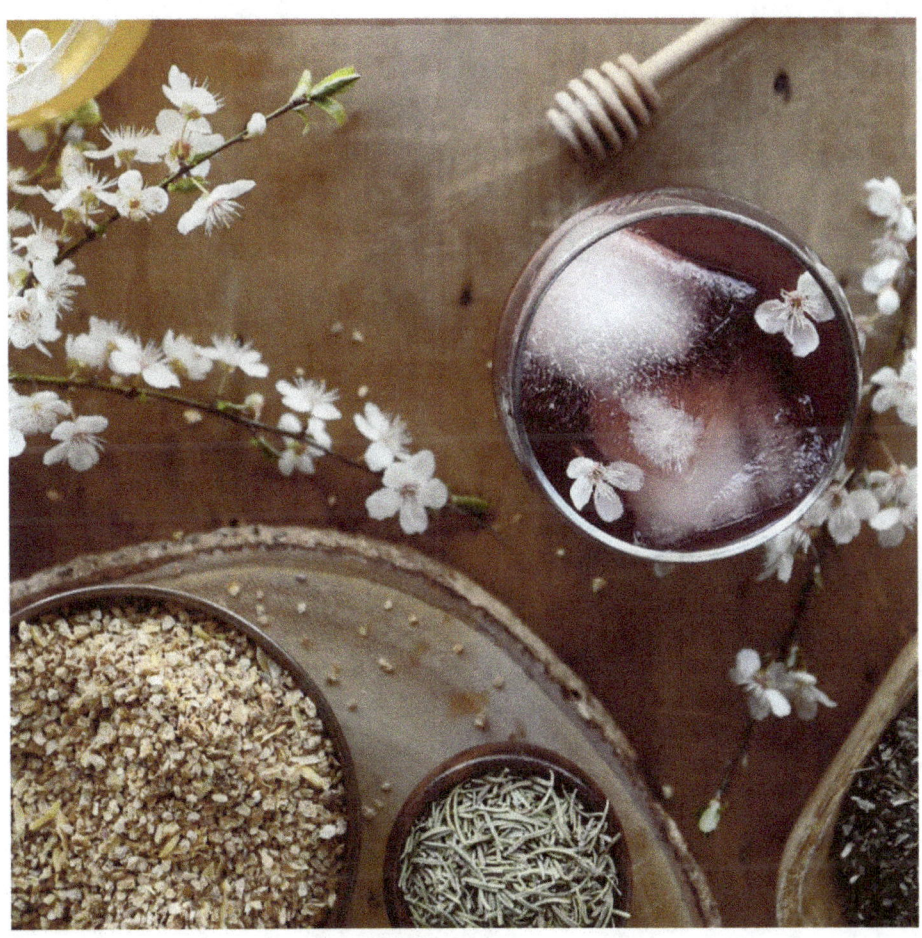

HOW TO ENJOY YOUR OXYMELS

When you've made your first amazing oxymel, try adding some to warm water as a comforting drink to pull you through the sniffle season. Or, use a splash or two to flavor bubbly water on a hot summer day for a refreshing boost. You also might find you like it as a topping on pancakes or added to a vinaigrette for a garden salad.

OUR FAVORITE HERBS FOR OXYMELS

- elion
- Elderberries and elderflowers
- Garlic
- Lemon balm
- Hyssop
- Nettle
- Tulsi (Holy Basil): Rama, Krishna, or Vana
- Rosehips
- Turmeric
- Basil
- Elecampane
- Garlic
- Mullein
- Lemon Peel
- Thyme
- Oregano
- Rosemary

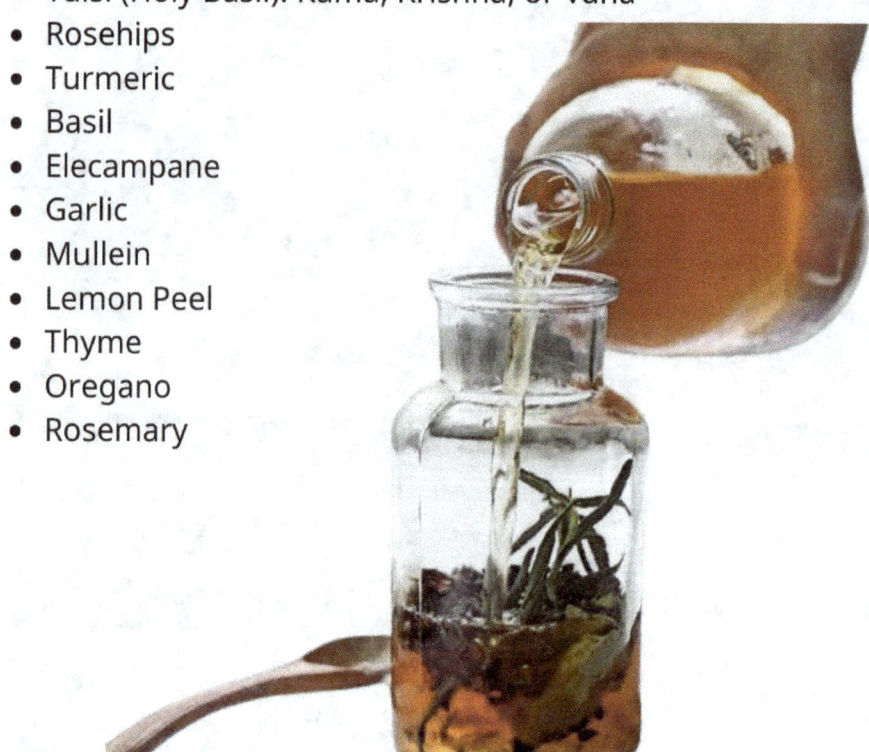

Pro Tips

- Remember, babies under 1 year of age should NEVER be given raw honey—no oxymels for the wee ones!
- I like to use local wildflower honey for its complexity of flavor, but if you want a more consistent and neutral flavor, use clover honey.
- You don't have to use raw apple cider vinegar, but many people believe it brings with it added health benefits. And it is excellent to use in making an alcohol-free extract.

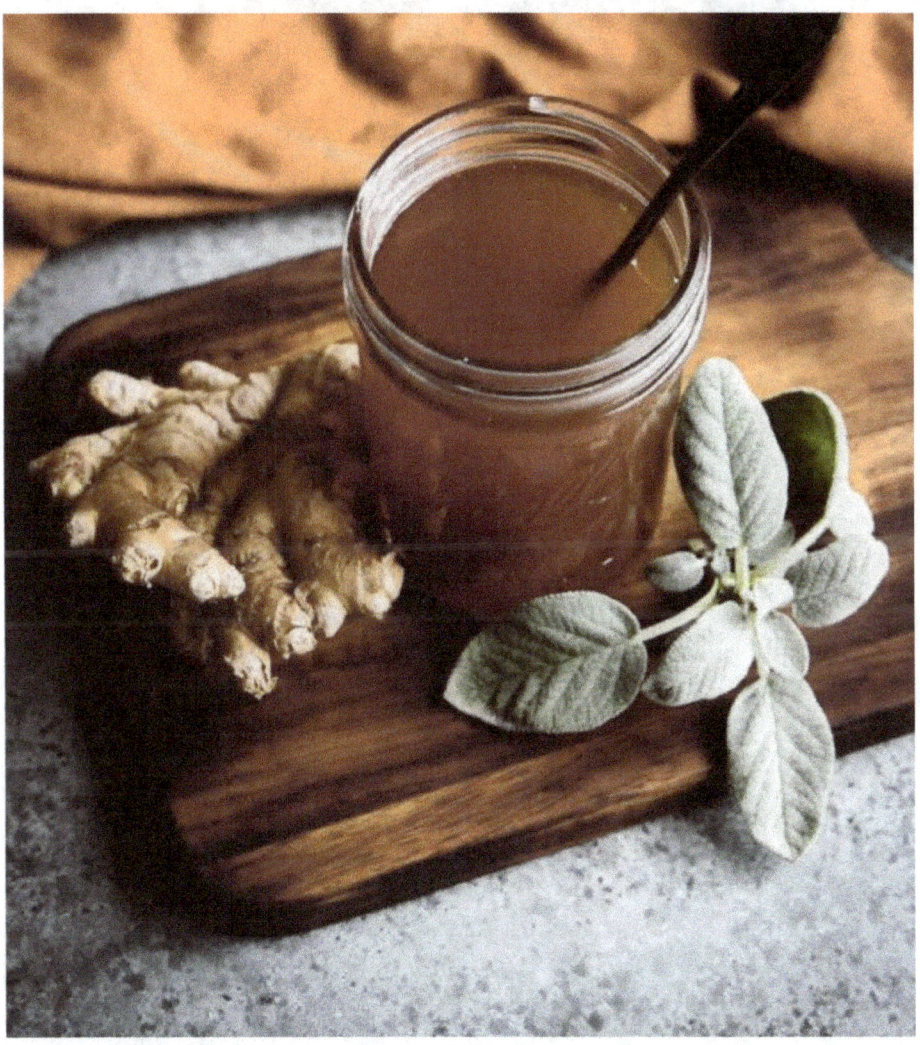

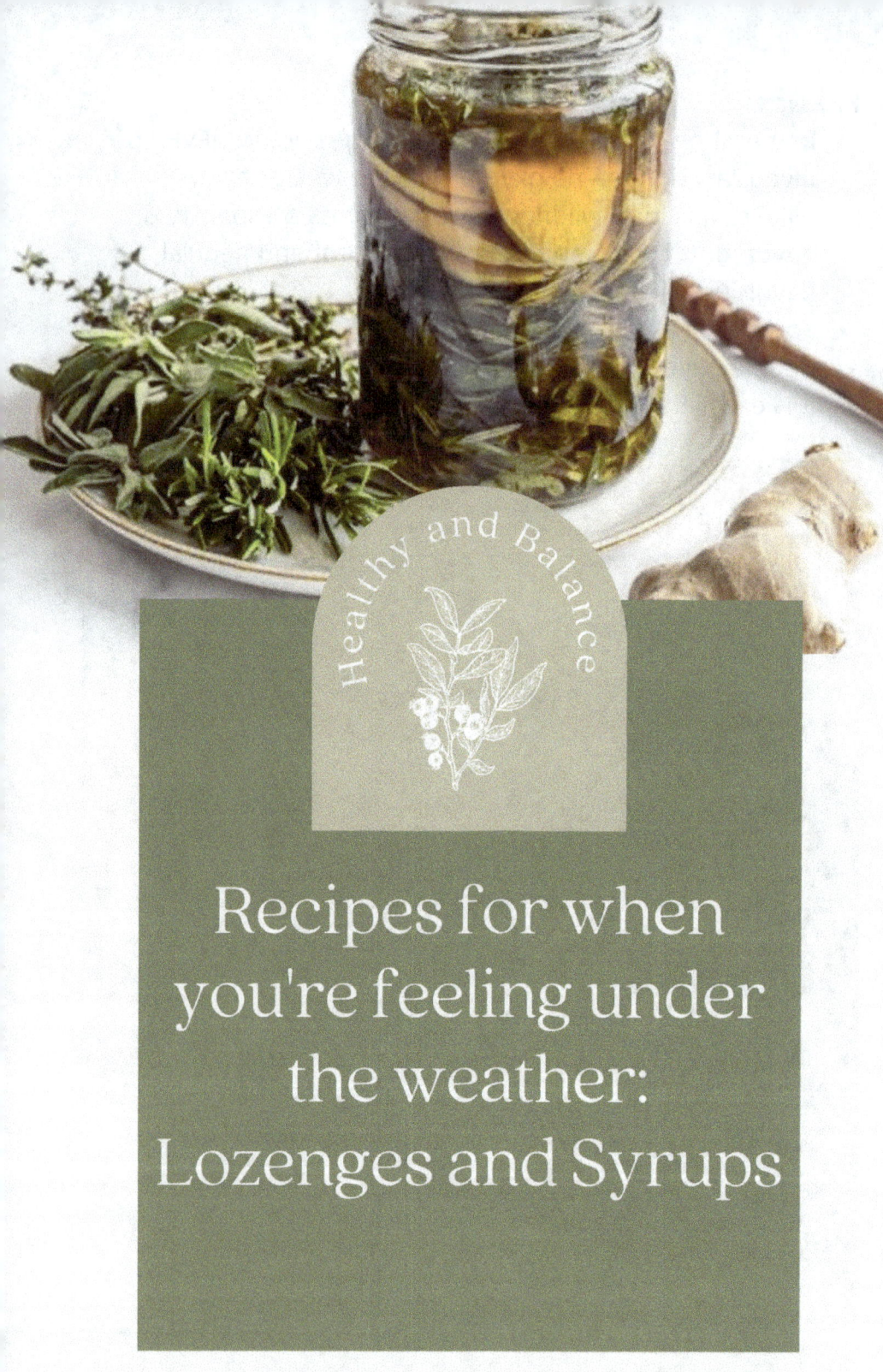

Healthy and Balance

Recipes for when you're feeling under the weather: Lozenges and Syrups

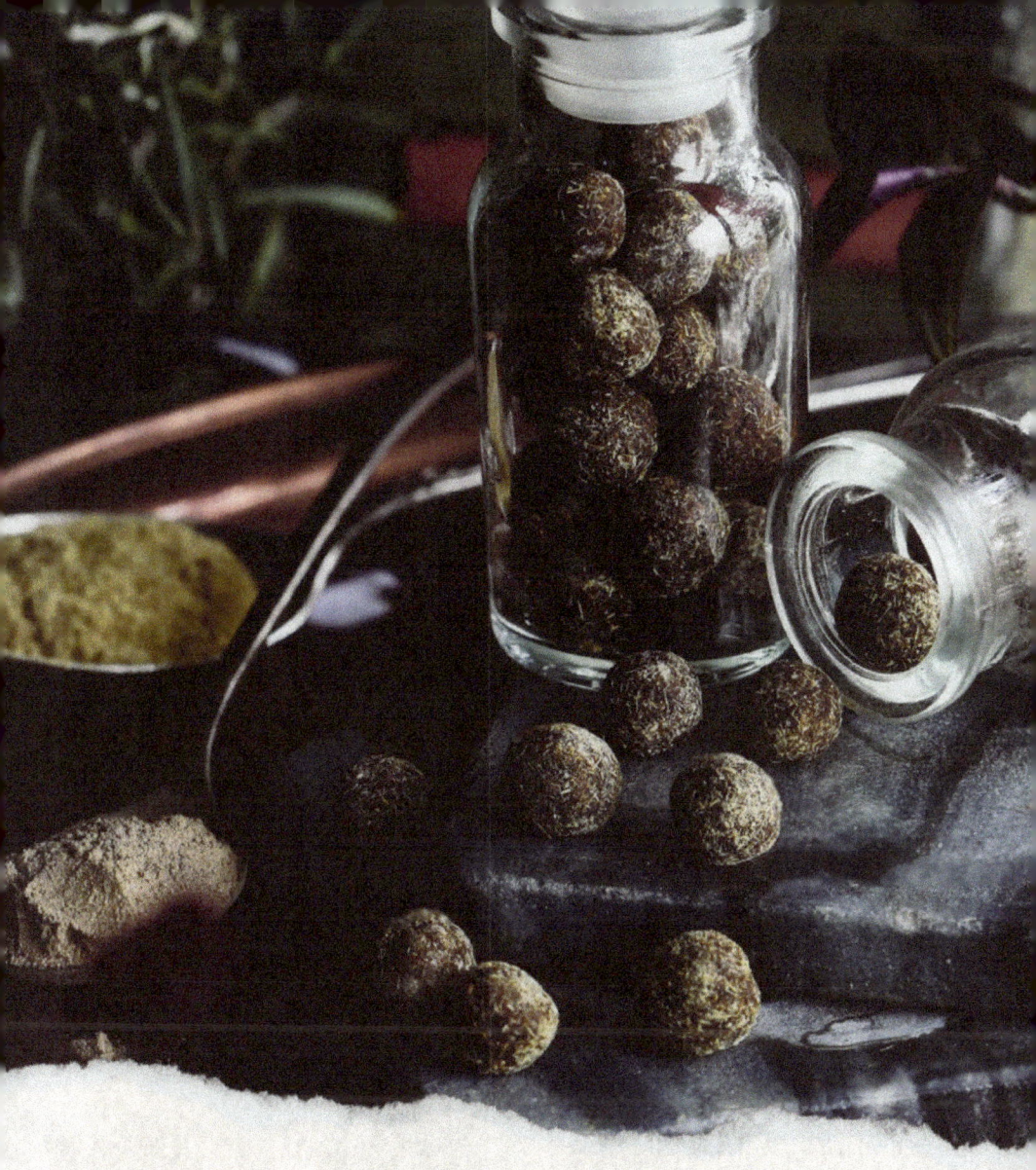

MAKING HOMEMADE
HERBAL LOZENGES

Stand beneath a blooming linden tree, and chances are you will slowly become aware of an almost unbelievable event taking place. The tree will be so alive with the hum and buzz of happy honeybees so absorbed in their harvest, they may very well bounce right off of you! An 80-year-old tree near my home presents a nearly surreal experience under her widespread, blooming boughs.

LINDEN LEAF & FLOWER POWDER

Linden, also known as tilia, is a gentle, generous herb definitely worth getting to know. Many people find it calming, relaxing, and even mood-lifting. It has expectorant action, so it may help to clear some of the seasonal grossness that can block us up during pollen season. It is also diaphoretic, slightly raising the body temperature and encouraging perspiration, which can be useful during those "under-the-weather" days and making it a useful year-round remedy. Plus, the scent is delicious! Linden can be enjoyed as a tea, in a nourishing herbal infusion, as an extract, or in capsules.

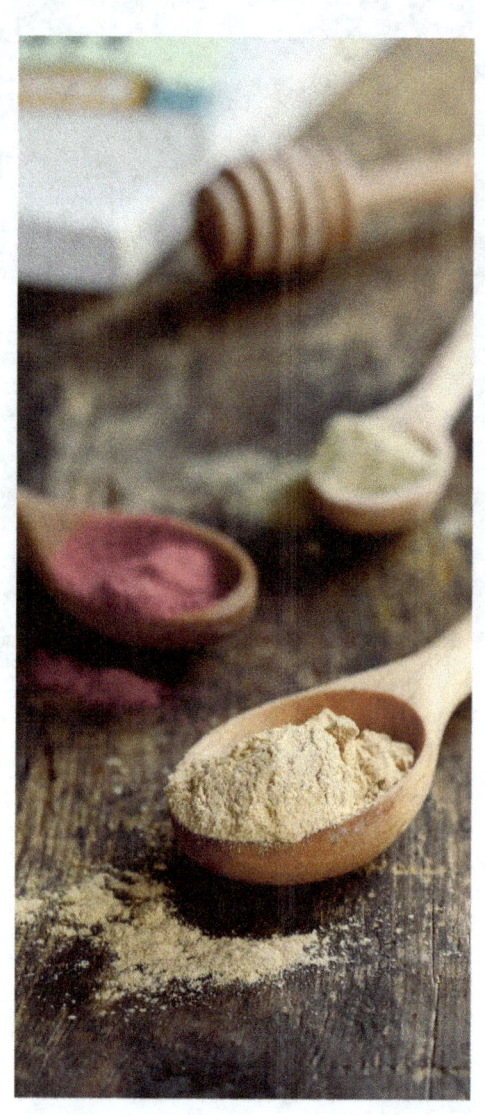

HERBAL LOZENGES

Herbal lozenges, also known as herbal pastilles or herbal tablets, are a method of consuming an herb without needing to prepare a food or beverage in which to incorporate it. They are quick to make, convenient to take, and easy to keep on hand in a desk drawer or handbag! Herbalists enjoy making lozenges because they also allow us to taste and consume the whole herb, as opposed to just the components that can be extracted or infused. Like other herbal preparations, they are adjustable to your unique needs and herbal preferences.

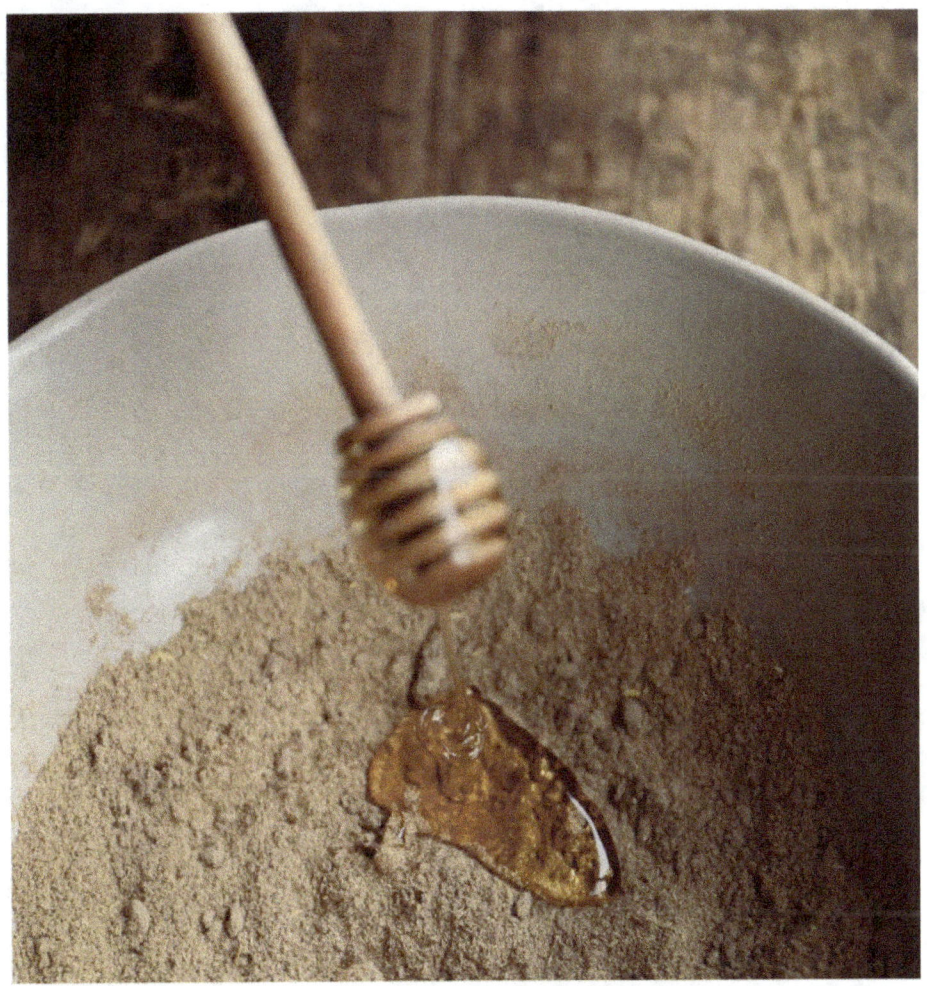

Homemade Linden & Honey Herbal Lozenges

Active time: 15 minutes

Ingredients

- 8 parts hand-ground organic linden leaf and flower
- 2 parts other herb powder (for flavor) such as organic orange peel powder, organic beet root powder, organic lavandin flower powder, or organic hibiscus flower powder
- 3 parts raw, local honey
- 1 part other liquid such as tincture (I like organic elderberry extract) or elixir (like ginger syrup)

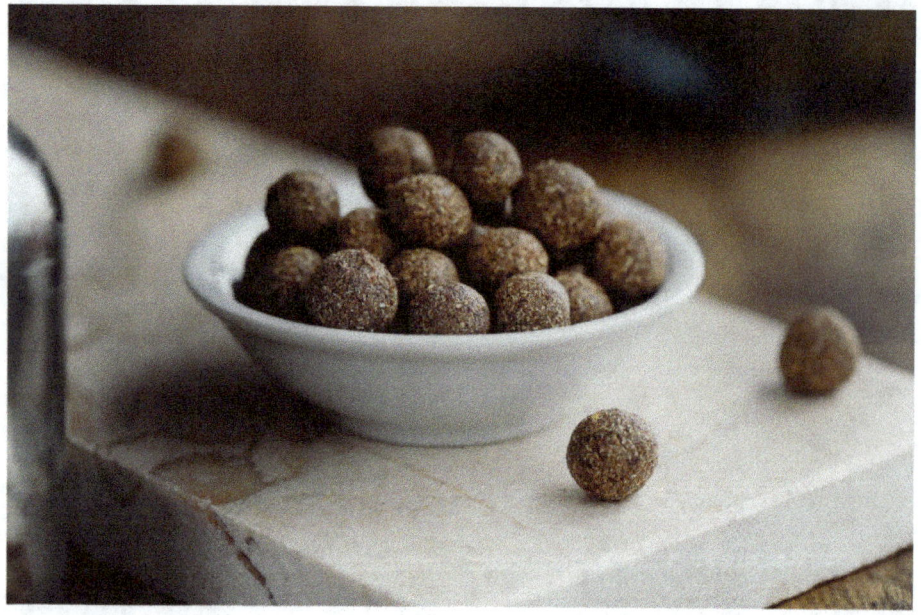

Directions

- Using a mortar and pestle, grind linden to the consistency of course powder.
- Mix ground linden with other dry ingredients.
- Slowly add wet ingredients. It should come together like a firm play dough.

- If the dough is too wet or sticky to work with, add more linden powder a little at a time until it reaches the desired consistency.
- If the dough is too dry and won't hold together, add small amounts of honey or liquid of choice until it is right.
- Form the dough into small, quarter-inch balls or disks.
- Dust with a finishing herbal powder such as orange powder or hibiscus powder.

Pro Tips

- If this is your first time making these lozenges, start with a teaspoon for each part (you'll need 10 teaspoons of herb total).
- If the dough is moist, flatten the balls (so they dry quickly) or roll the dough into a log and slice off "coins."

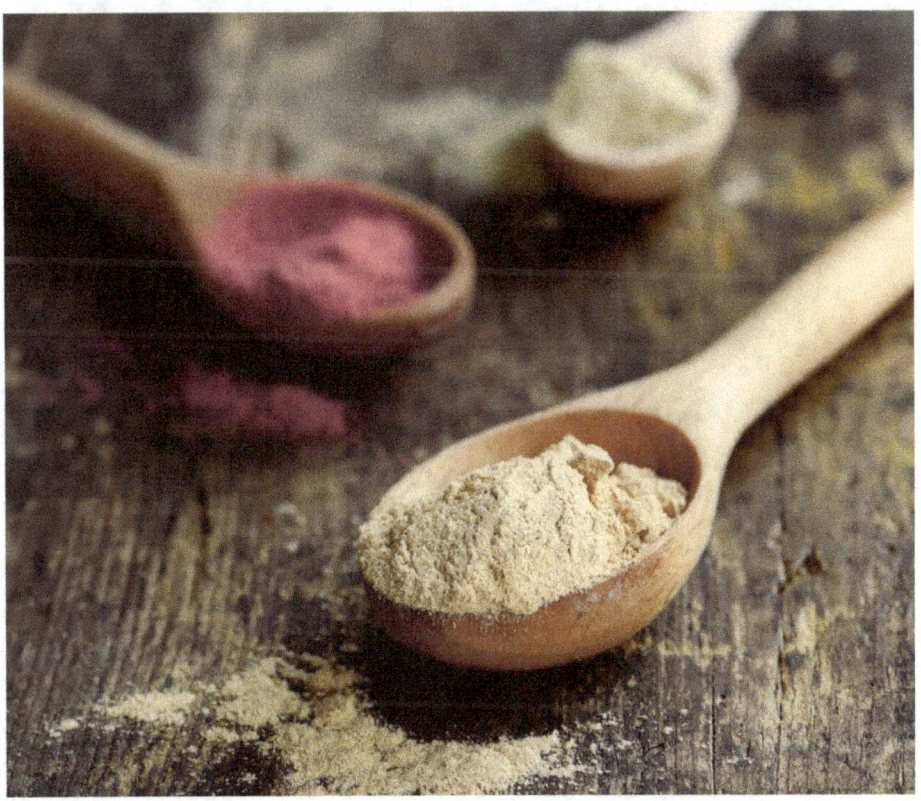

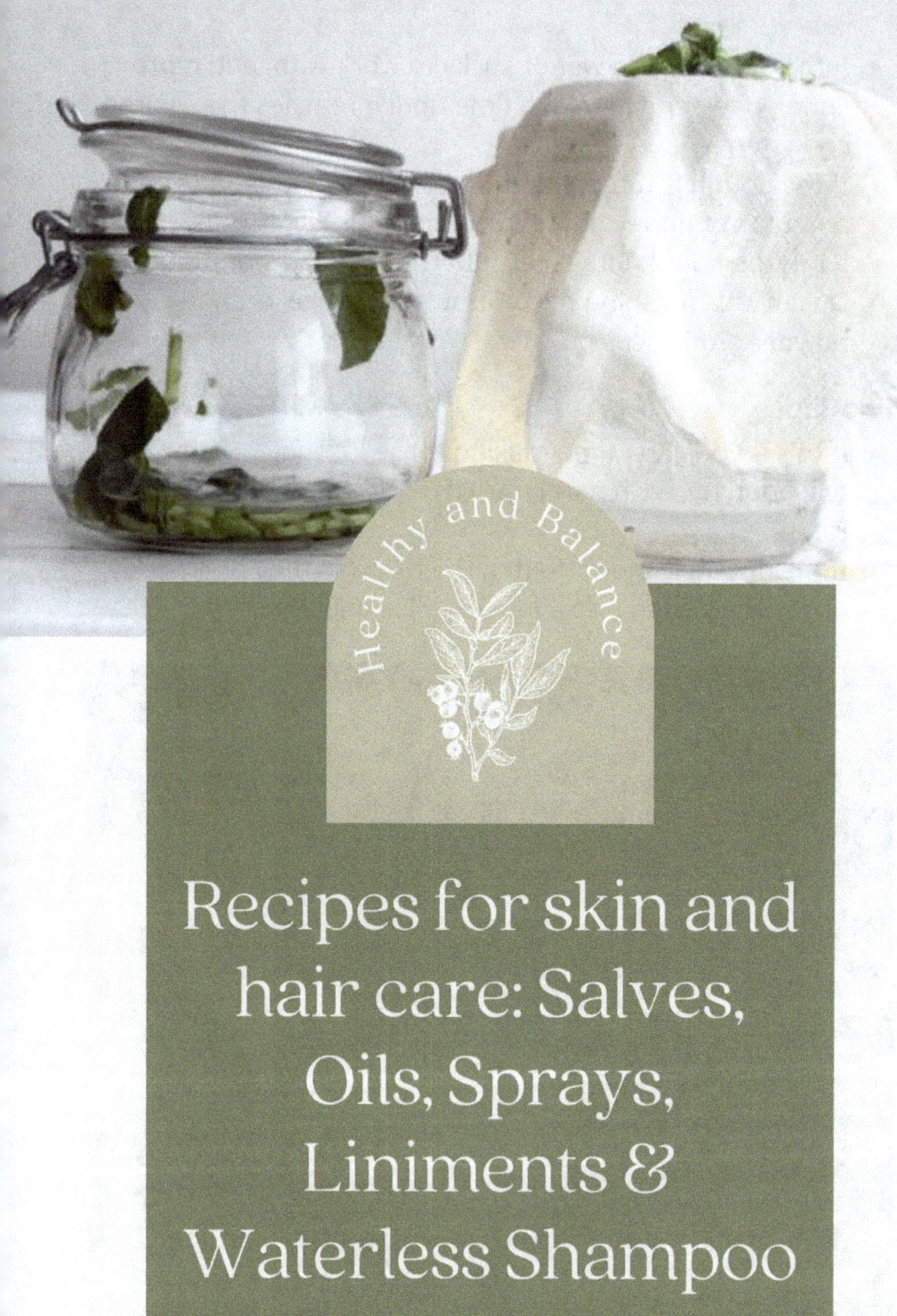

Recipes for skin and hair care: Salves, Oils, Sprays, Liniments & Waterless Shampoo

Healthy and Balance

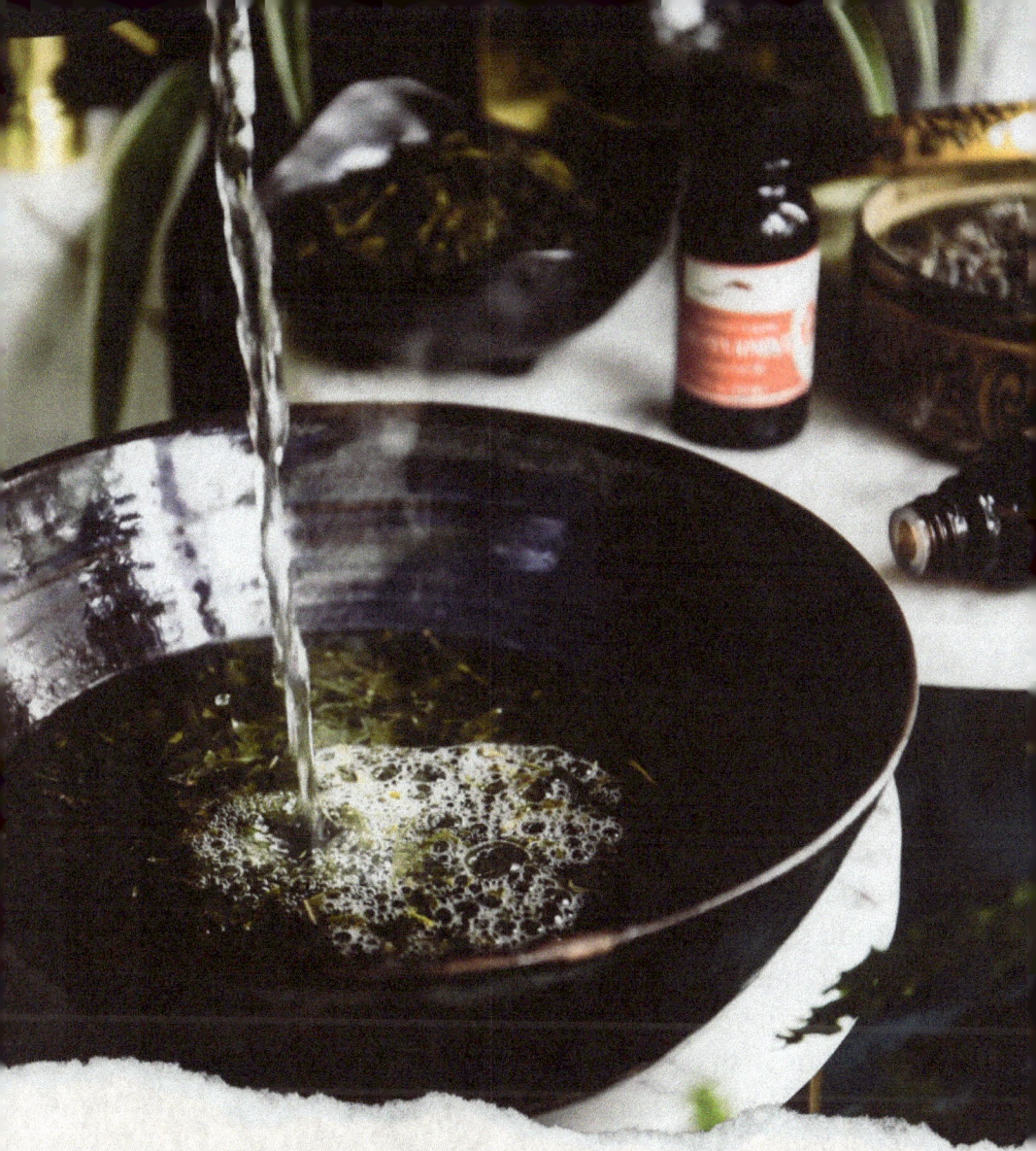

HOW TO MAKE HERBAL SALVES

How to Make Herbal Salves

Herbal salves are such a simple, effective, and useful way to take in herbal goodness! They can easily be slipped into a purse, pocket, or first aid kit. Although semi-solid at room temperature, salves soften once applied to the skin, making them less messy than oils. They also make great gifts and are an easy and approachable way to introduce newbies to the power of herbs. Plus, salves can be crafted for a wide variety of topical uses. The addition of beeswax will protect, soothe, and nourish your skin.

Part 1: Make Herb-Infused Oil

To make a salve, first craft your herb-infused oil(s). This can take anywhere from about a day to several weeks, depending on the method used. You can also purchase infused herbal oils if you're short on time or wish to skip the process of infusing the oil yourself. We recommend using only dried herbs in your infusions, as the lack of moisture content in the plant material can keep spoilage at bay.

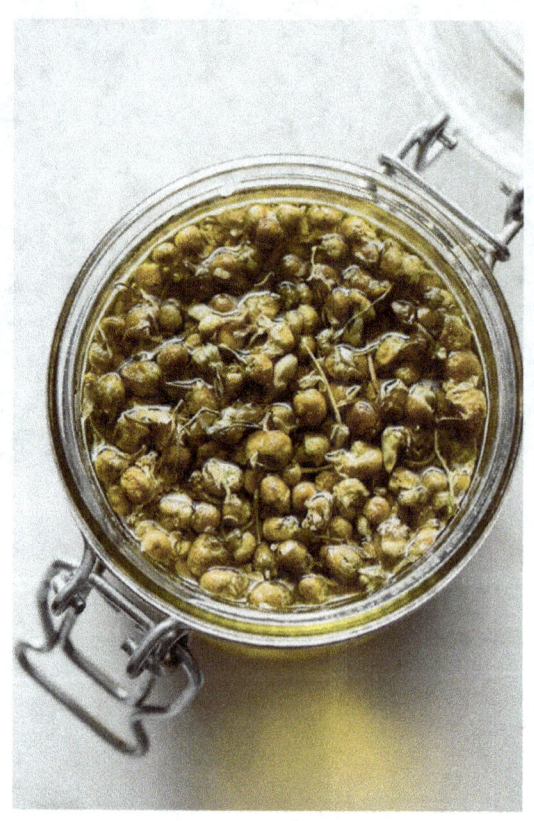

Part 2: Make Your Salve

Once you've created your herbal oil, you're just a few simple steps away from your finished salve! See our basic salve recipe below, and follow along with herbal educator and author Maria Noël Groves for a comprehensive video how-to demonstration!
Makes 5 ounces.

Ingredients
- 1 oz. beeswax (use carnauba wax for a vegan salve)
- 4 oz. herbal infused oil(s) of your choice (choose one or a combination)
- 10-20 drops essential oil of choice (optional)

Directions
1. Wrap beeswax bar in an old towel. On a sturdy surface, use a hammer to break bar up into small chunks.
2. Place beeswax in a double boiler and gently warm over low heat until the beeswax melts.
3. Add herbal oils and stir over low heat until well-mixed.
4. Remove from heat and add the essential oil(s).
5. Quickly pour warm mixture into prepared tins, glass jars, or lip balm tubes and allow to cool completely.
6. Store in a cool location for 1 to 3 years.

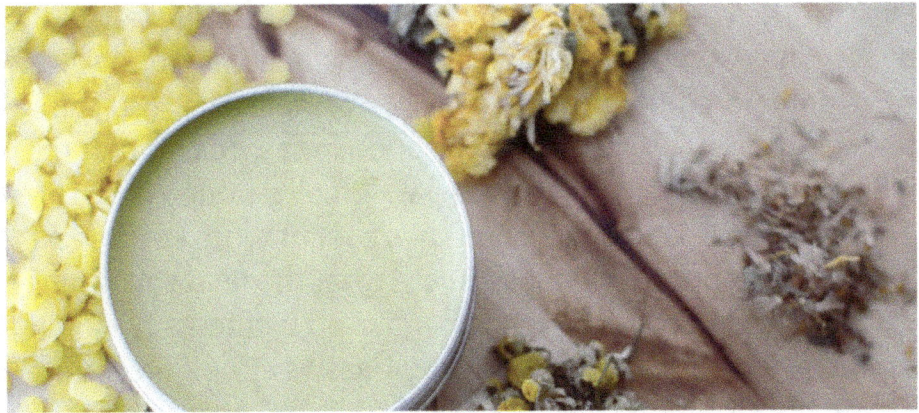

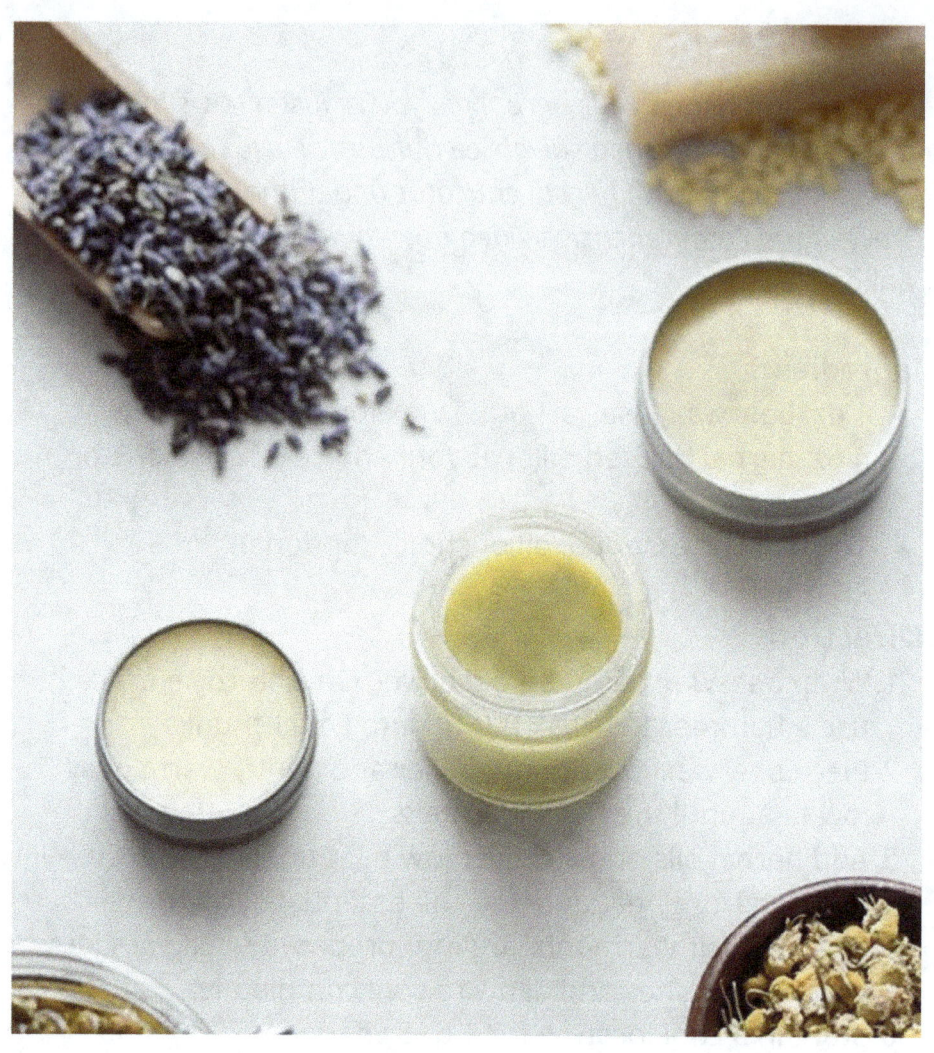

Pro tip: The consistency of salves can easily be adjusted depending on your preferences. Use less beeswax for a softer salve and more beeswax if you'd like a firmer salve. You can test the consistency by placing a spoon in the freezer before making your salve. When the beeswax melts, pour a little salve onto one of the cold spoons and place it back into the freezer for 1 to 2 minutes. This will simulate what the final consistency will be like. Once cooled, you can make adjustments by adding more oil (for a softer salve) or more beeswax (for a firmer salve).

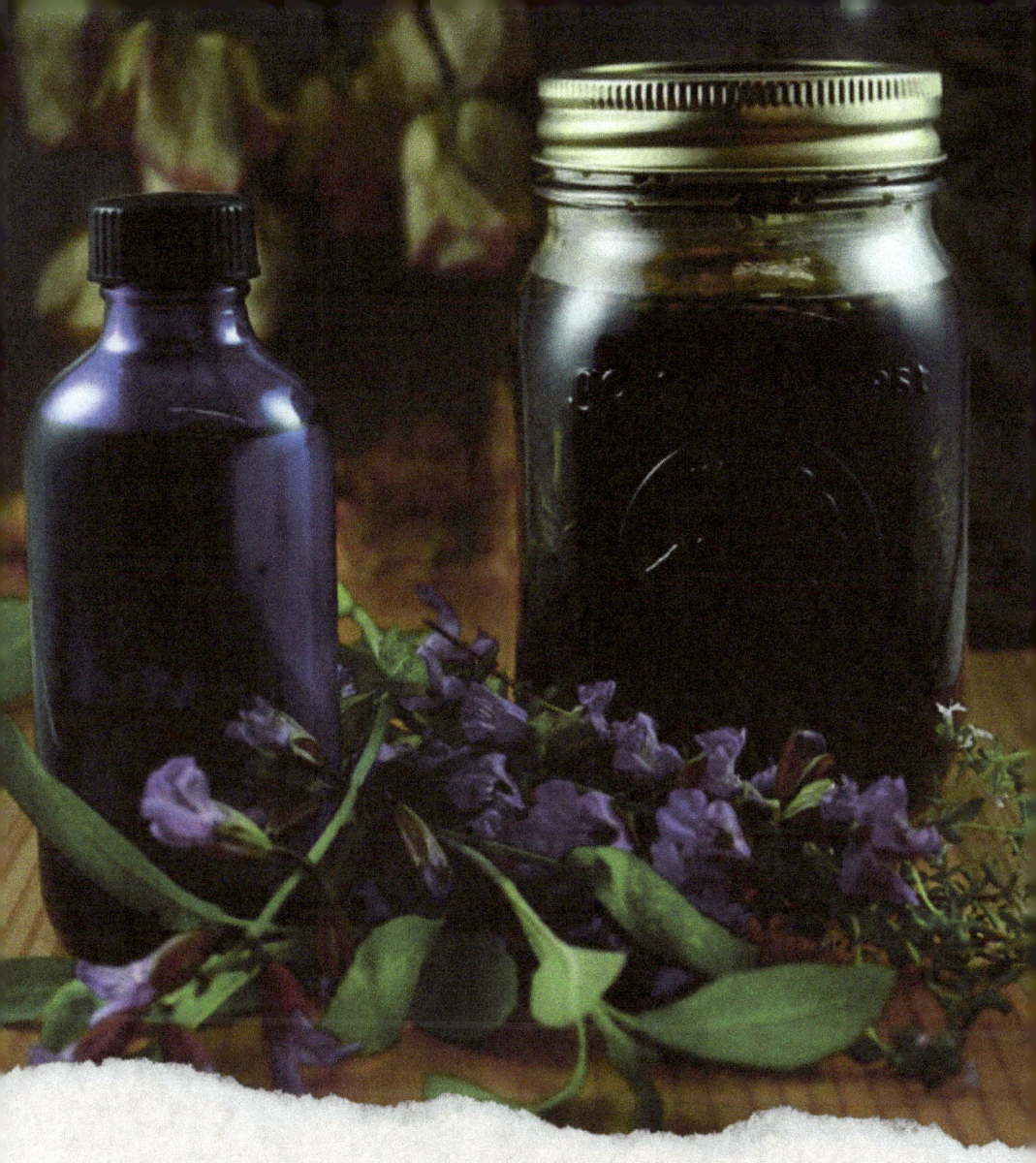

HERBAL LINIMENTS

Simple to make, herbal liniments are a great element for any home first aid cabinet!

Liniments can be formulated to warm or cool. Warming herbs like black pepper, cayenne, or ginger can be added to help support normal blood circulation and assist with everyday stiffness. Herbs like peppermint or menthol crystals are useful for general cooling.

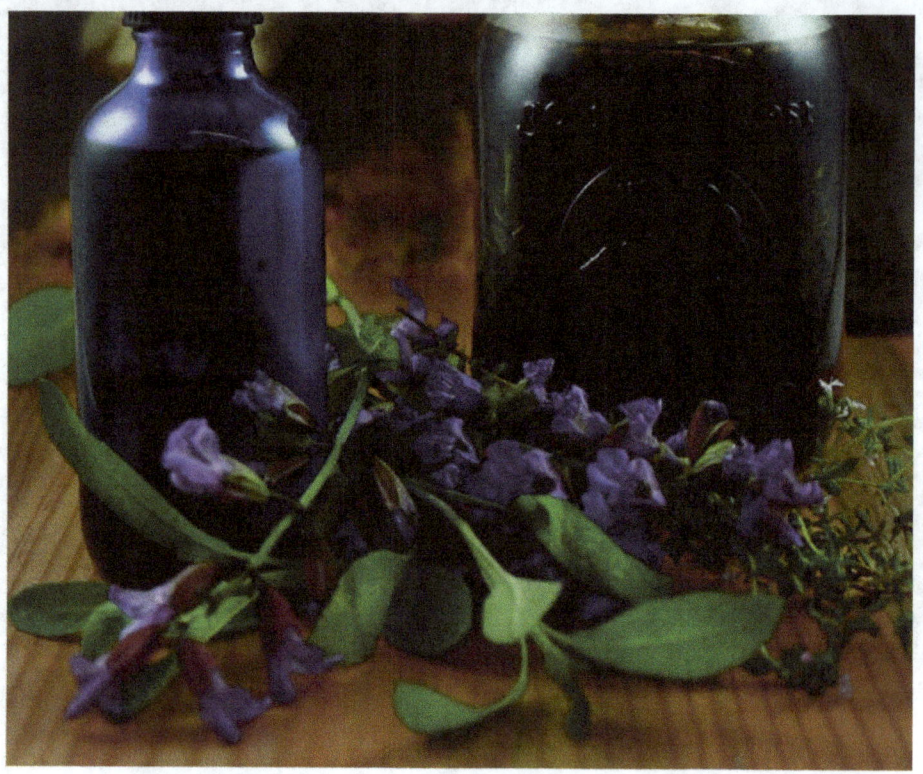

Basic Herbal Liniment

This recipe provides the basic guidelines for making herbal liniments and is completely customizable.

Ingredients

- Rubbing Alcohol or other menstruum of choice. *See note below.

- Fresh or dried herbs. Popular choices are: arnica, black pepper, calendula, cayenne, chamomile, comfrey, echinacea, eucalyptus, ginger, goldenseal, lavender, myrrh, oregano, oregon grape root, peppermint, rosemary, St. John's wort, thyme, and yarrow.
- Optional additions: menthol crystals and/or essential oil(s) of choice.

Directions
- Place herbs in a clean glass jar. If using fresh herbs, chop them first.
- Cover thoroughly with rubbing alcohol or other menstruum of choice, and cap with a tight-fitting lid.
- Place the jar in a warm area and shake daily or as often as possible.
- After 4-6 weeks, strain the herbs out using cheesecloth.
- If desired, add Menthol crystals (they will dissolve in alcohol) and/or essential oil(s). Pour the liniment into dark glass bottles.
- Make sure to label the liniment for "External Use Only".

When properly stored in a cool dark place, the liniment will keep almost indefinitely.

To use: gently rub onto skin and allow to evaporate. Be careful not to rub too hard or vigorously as this can cause irritation.

Note: Rubbing alcohol is typically used to make liniments because it extracts the herbal constituents and rapidly penetrates and evaporates from the skin. You could also use Vodka, Witch Hazel Extract, or Vinegar as a solvent. Basically, you'll need a menstruum to extract the properties of the herbs which will absorb quickly and deeply to penetrate skin. If alcohol alone is too harsh or drying on your skin, try mixing it with Witch Hazel Extract or Vinegar until you find a medium that works for you.

Kloss Liniment

Available in Rosemary Gladstar's book Medicinal Herbs: A Beginners Guide, this very old and strong recipe was first published by the famous herbalist Dr. Jethro Kloss in his classic book Back to Eden in 1939. Kloss's liniment is useful for helping occasional sore muscles. Instead of Goldenseal, you can also substitute Chaparral or Oregon Grape Root.

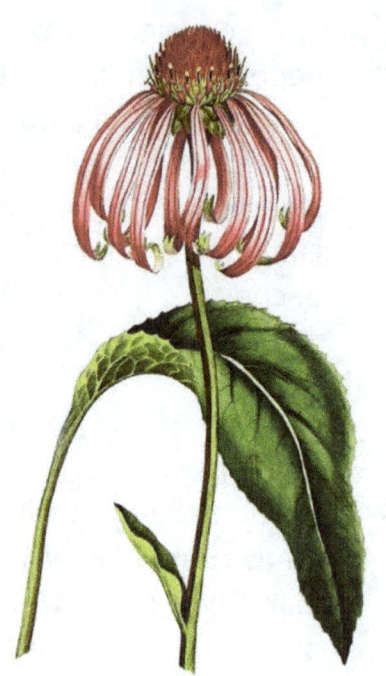

Ingredients
- 1 oz. organic echinacea powder
- 1 oz. organically grown goldenseal powder (may substitute chaparral or Oregon grape root)
- 1 oz. wildharvested myrrh powder
- ¼ oz. organic cayenne powder
- 1 pint Rubbing Alcohol

Directions
- Place the powder in a jar and cover with rubbing alcohol (a food-grade alcohol can be used, but rubbing alcohol seems to work best), leaving a good 2-inch margin above the herbs.
- Cover with a tight-fitting lid.
- Place the mixture in a warm location and let it sit for 4 weeks.
- Strain and rebottle. Label the bottle clearly for "External Use Only".

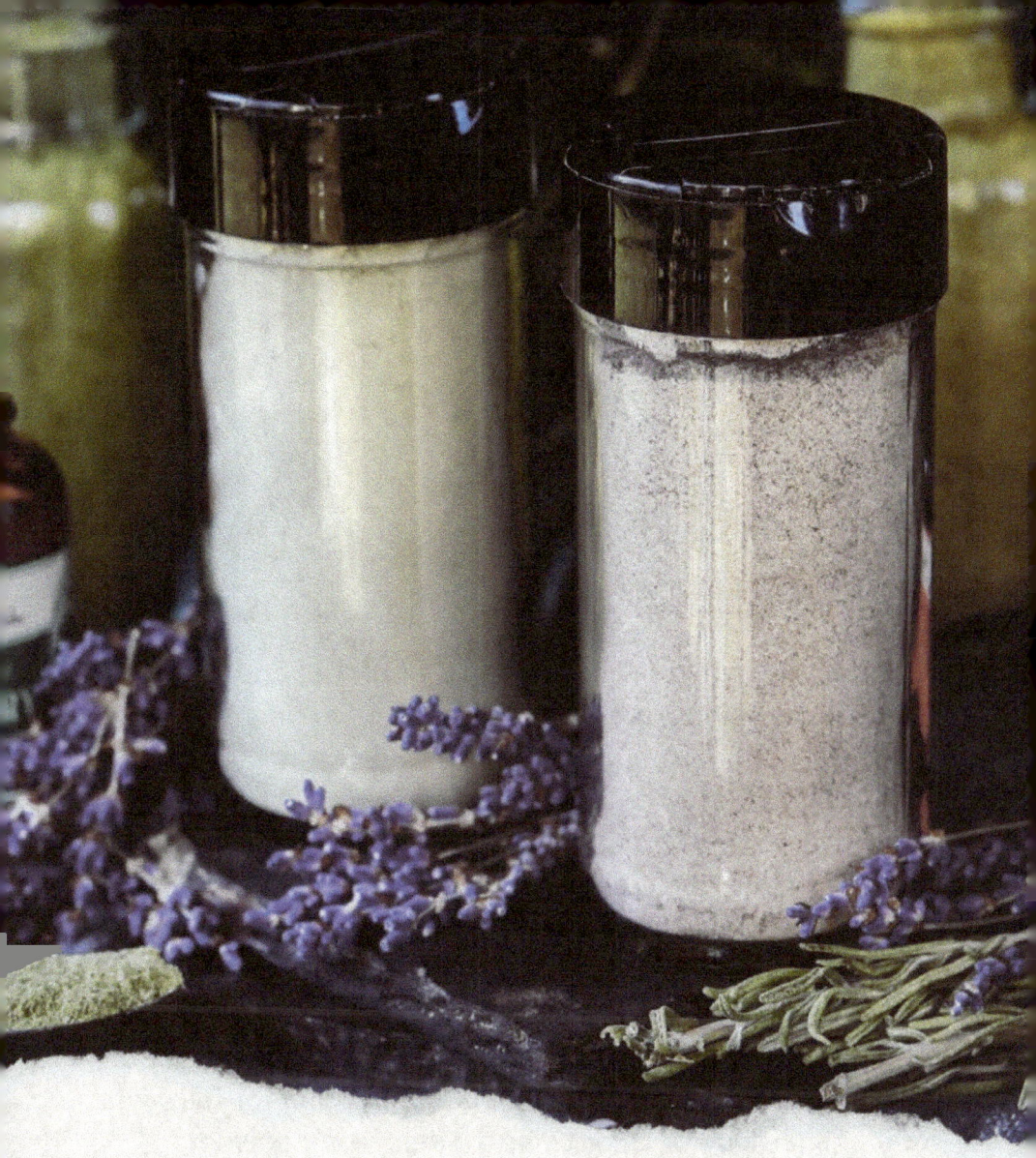

DIY DRY SHAMPOO RECIPES FOR DARK & LIGHT HAIR

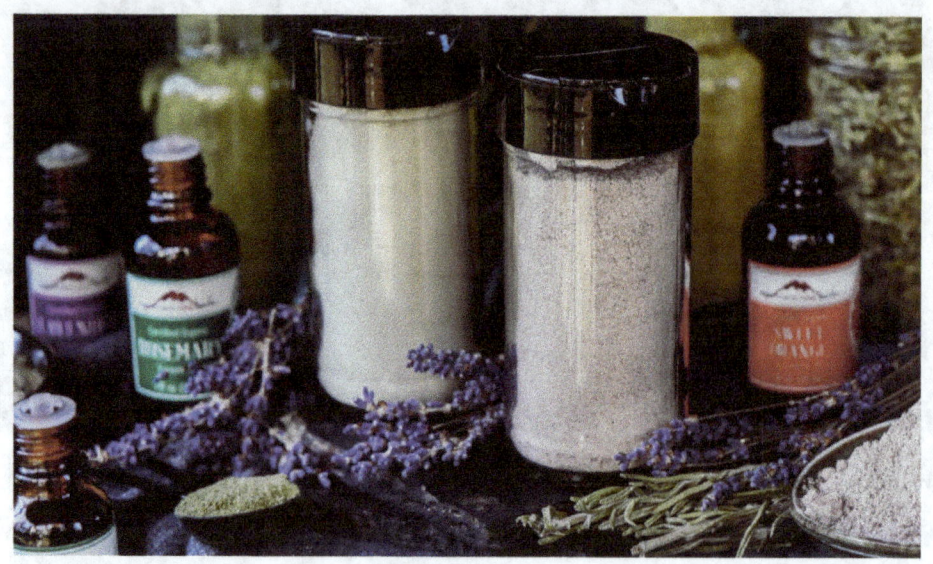

There has been a lot of buzz lately around DIY and natural hair care. In the previous weeks, we've shared no-poo recipes, DIY hair rinses, and fermented rice water treatments. A perfect pairing to all those homemade hair care products is having a dry shampoo to get you in between "washes."

Dry "shampoos" are created to work without water, and there has been a long history of people using powdered herbs, grains, and natural cosmetic clays to remove excess oil and dirt build-up. These ingredients naturally absorb oils and can then be brushed out without causing damage to the hair or scalp. Dry shampoos can also be a good option for folks who want to shampoo once or twice a week, using powders between washings to keep hair fresh, full, and manageable. They also come in handy when packing for camping trips and outdoor festivals!

We've created two different powders, one dry shampoo for dark hair (made with cocoa or carob powder) and another for lighter hair colors, but you can adjustment ingredients to suit your needs. Both shampoo blends are built around a base of organic tapioca powder, a super lightweight starch that becomes pretty much invisible once applied.

Homemade Dry Shampoo Recipes

Ingredients
ROSEMARY COCOA SHAMPOO POWDER (FOR DARKER HAIR)

- 1/2 cup organic organic tapioca powder or arrowroot powder
- 1/4 cup baking soda
- 1/2 cup organic cacao powder or organic carob powder
- 1 Tbsp. organic rosemary powder
- 1 Tbsp. organic oatstraw powder
- 10 drops each organic rosemary and organic bergamot essential oils

LAVENDER & SWEET ORANGE SHAMPOO POWDER (FOR LIGHTER HAIR)

- 1/2 cup organic organic tapioca powder or arrowroot powder
- 1/2 cup French green cosmetic clay
- 1 Tbsp. organic oatstraw powder
- 1 Tbsp. organic lavender flower powder
- 1 Tbsp. organic chamomile powder
- 10 drops each organic sweet orange and organic lavender essential oils

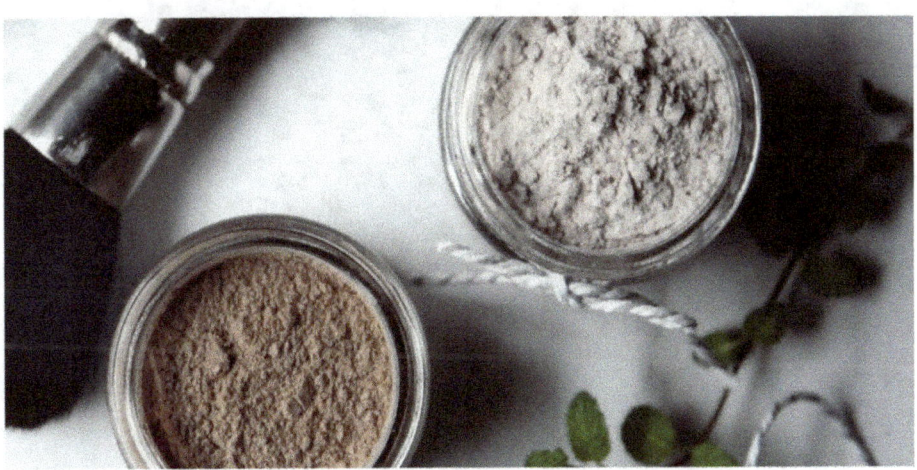

Directions

- Mix all the ingredients together and stir well to combine.
- Transfer finished blend into a dry container and store away from moisture (to reduce clumping).
- Use as necessary.

How to Use Dry Shampoo

- Shake or sprinkle powdered shampoo blend along the crown of the head, working through the scalp and hair to pick up any excess oils or debris.
- Depending on the texture and thickness of your hair, either brush or shake well to remove the excess.
- It's best to do this right before bed or before you get dressed so you don't wind up with any powder residue on your clothes.
- You can also drape your shoulders with a towel to keep the powder off your clothes.

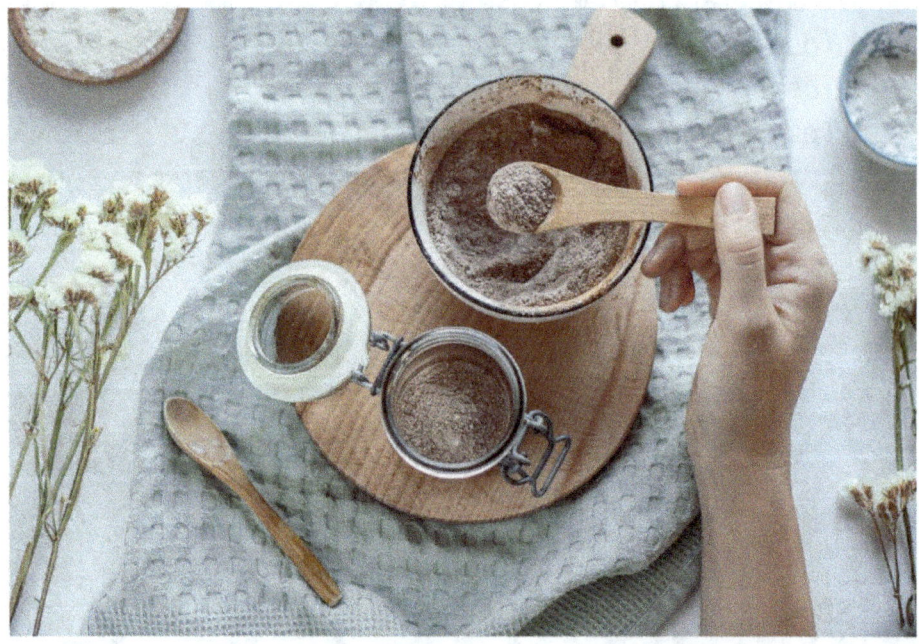

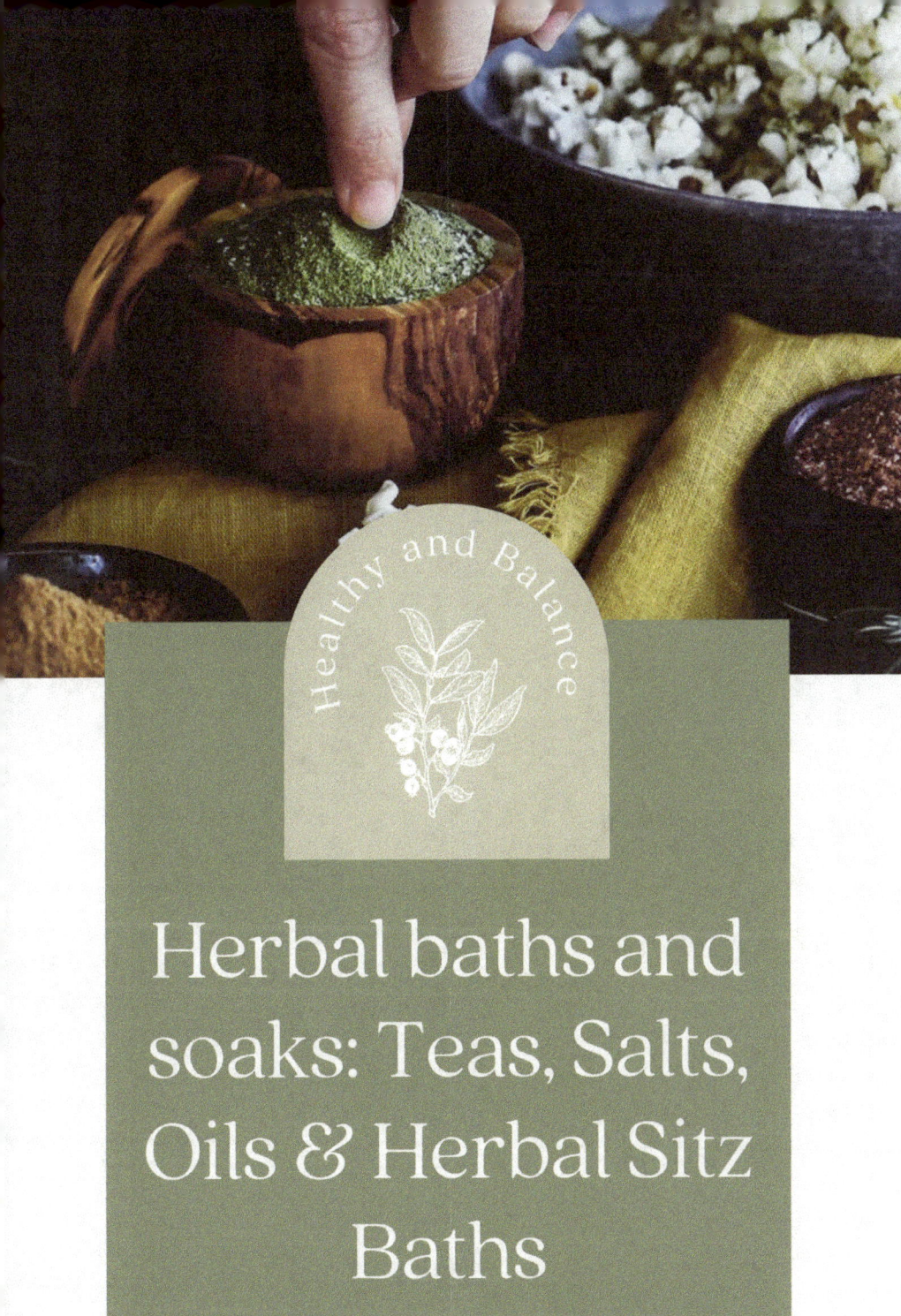

Herbal baths and soaks: Teas, Salts, Oils & Herbal Sitz Baths

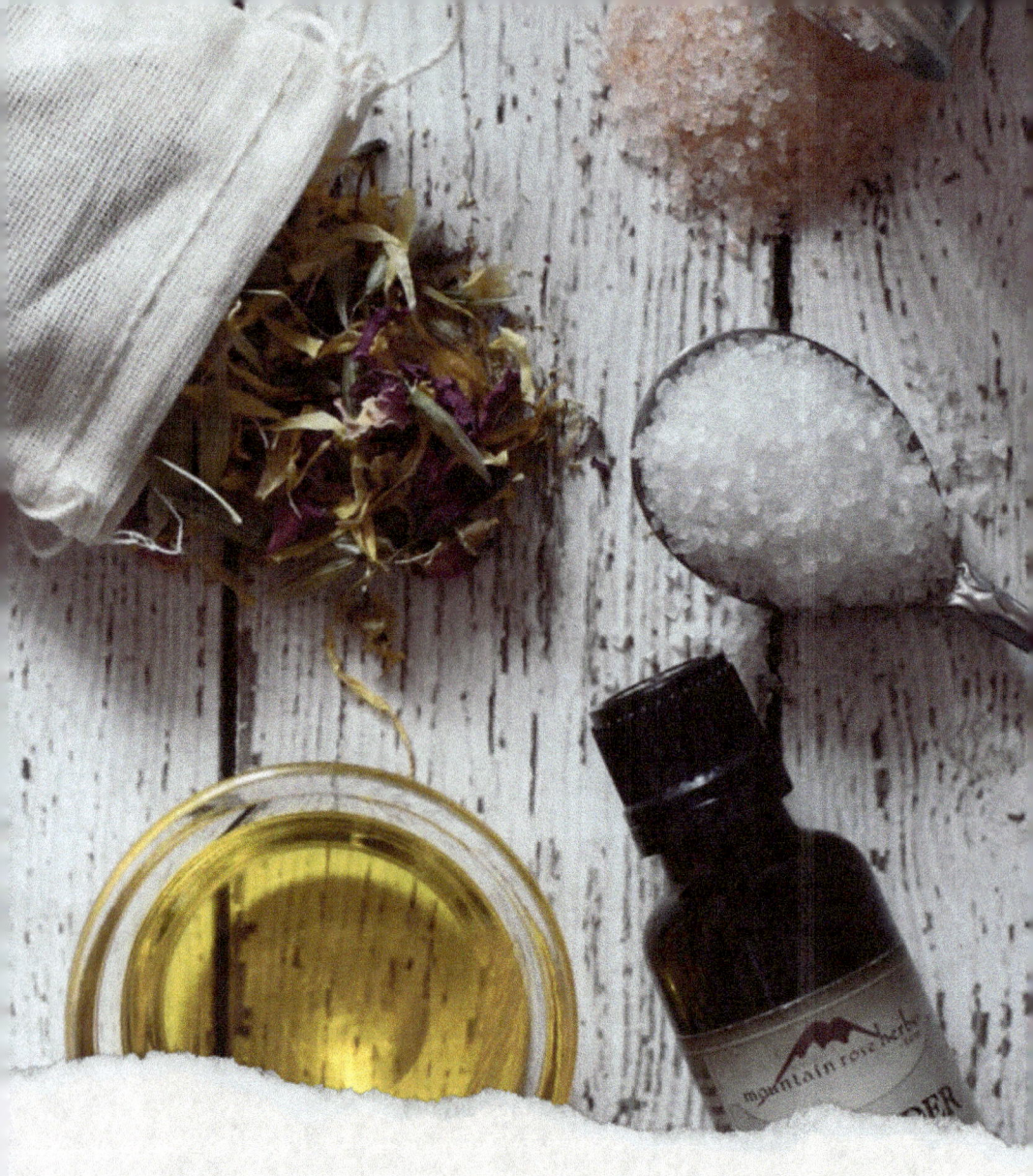

MAKING HERBAL BATH SALTS, OILS & TEA SOAKS

Whether submerged in a forest-nestled hot spring, floating on the surface of a high mountain lake, or luxuriating in the warm lapping ocean, water is an essential element for physical and emotional well-being. Taking time to bathe in the ancient restorative power that water offers can be transformative, and sometimes this simple pleasure is the perfect medicine for whatever ails us. The sensuous comfort water provides connects us back to both our bodies and the Earth's beauty.

Bath Salt Soak

Ingredients
- 2/3 cup salt of your choice: Himalayan pink salt, epsom salt, or coarse sea salt
- 1/4 cup baking soda
- 10-25 drops organic essential oil of your choice: lavender, spruce, rosemary, geranium, peppermint, sweet orange, sandalwood, frankincense

Directions
1. Mix salt and baking soda together until combined.
2. Drip in the essential oil and stir well. Sprinkle 1/4 to 1/2 cup into your bath as hot water fills the tub.
3. Once dissolved, step in and soak your troubles away.

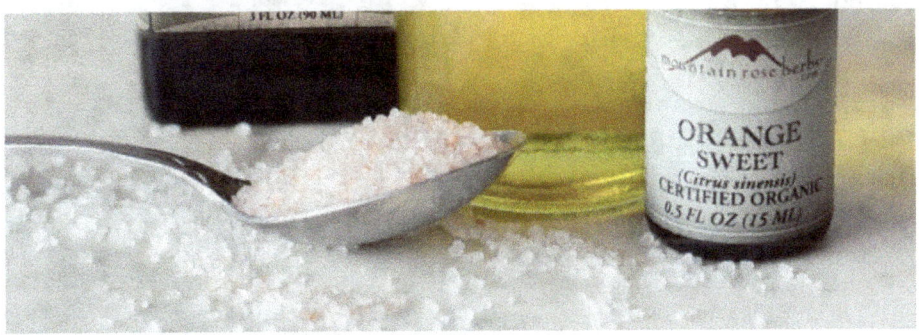

Aromatic Bath Oil

Ingredients
- 4 oz organic carrier oil
- 20 to 40 drops organic essential oil that's skin-friendly

Directions
1. Choose an organic carrier oil for your base such as jojoba, rosehip seed, kukui nut, or sweet almond oil.
2. Select an essential oil for your particular mood or physical need. If you want something relaxing, try lavender. If you want an uplifting scent, try sweet orange or geranium. Need to soothe the muscles? Try rosemary. (Be sure to research the essential oil you use, as some of them are safer to use than others in topical preparations.)
3. Slowly drip your essential oil into the bottle, tighten the cap, and roll between the palms of your hands to blend. A
4. Add 1/4 ounce of the oil blend to a filled tub and swirl throughout the water before getting in to soak. Be sure to keep the oil well dispersed as you bathe.

TIPS: For a sweet addition, try infusing your carrier oil base with an organic vanilla bean for two weeks before blending with essential oils. Also, a teaspoon of organic unrefined coconut oil melted into your bath water is lovely and an easy option!

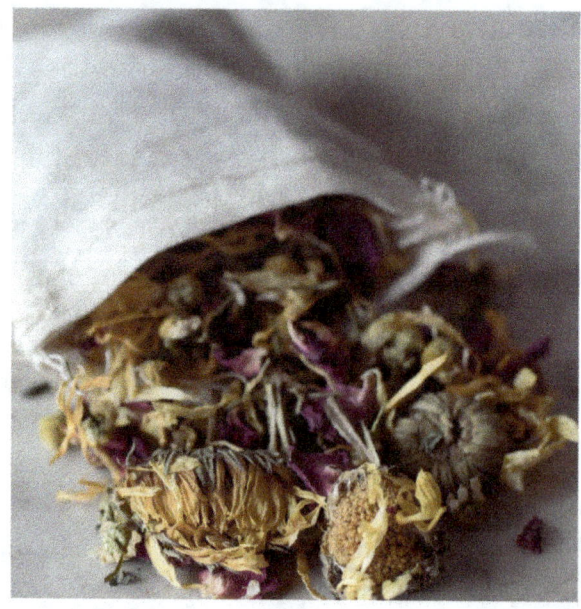

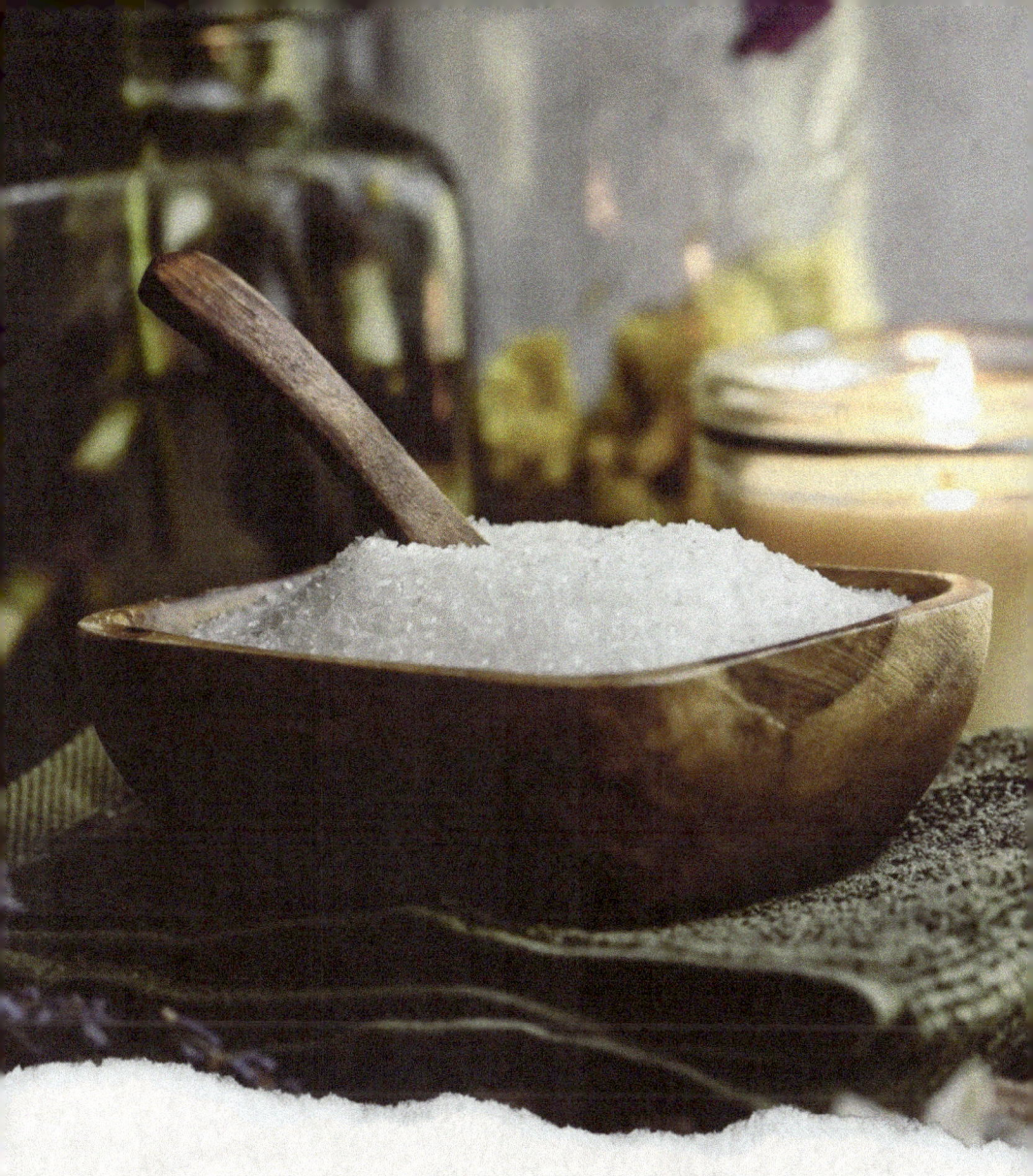

HOMEMADE HERBAL SITZ BATH

When I was a child, I was thrown from a horse and spent many years thereafter challenged by lower back and radiating leg pain. With time and maturity, as well as changes in my diet and appropriate exercise, I've put those pain-days behind me, but I've carried forward some of the best solutions that I learned from the experience. One of my favorites of these is the soothing comfort of an old-fashioned herbal sitz bath. Often used to relieve issues related to post-birth discomfort, etc., a sitz bath is also ideal for easing general lower-body soreness and fatigue.

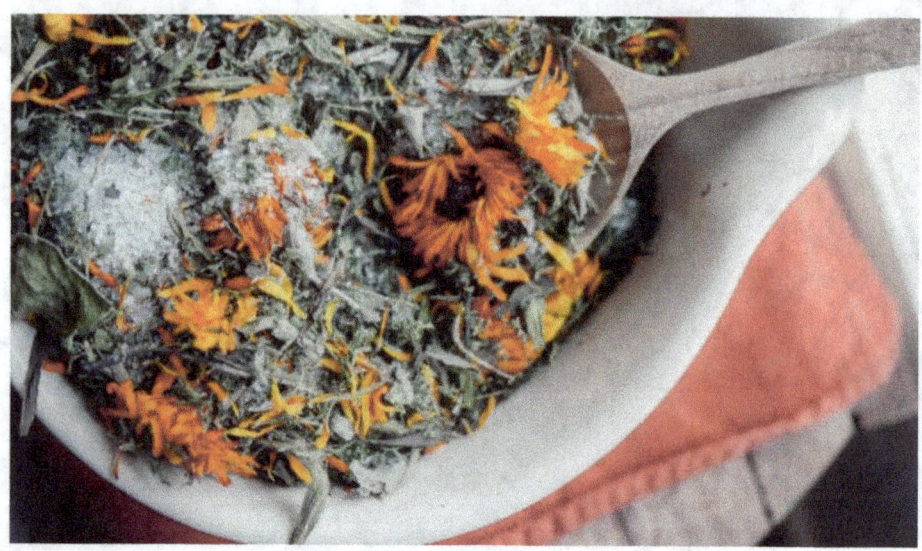

WHAT IS A SITZ BATH?

A sitz bath is a shallow bath in which you can add salts, herbs, and other ingredients to create a clean, warm, healing pool in which to sit. There are small tubs made specifically for this purpose, which are ideal for concentrating the salts and herbs where you need them most. However, when dealing with pain and fatigue that impacts the lower back and legs, a bathtub is the appropriate vessel.

The word "sitz" is from the German "sitzen"—no surprise, it means "to sit." There are other names for these short, soothing baths as well. My grandparents, for instance, prescribed taking a "hip bath" (water only up to the hips). I've also heard people call them a "salt soak," which makes sense because salts, particularly Epsom salt, are a ubiquitous ingredient in these little baths.

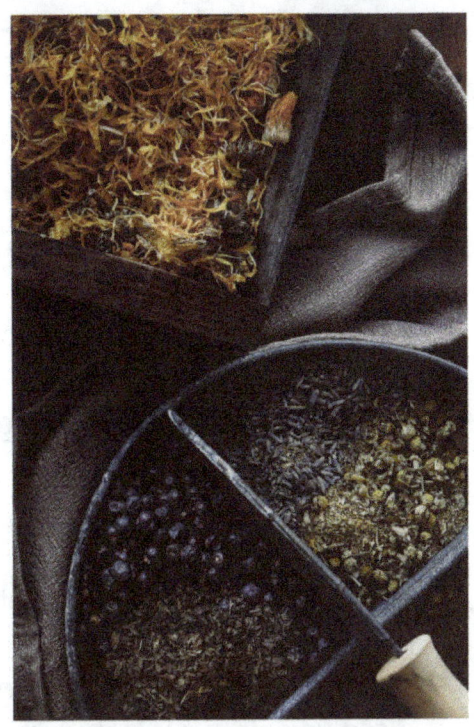

WHAT TO ADD TO A SITZ BATH

I make sitz baths much the way my grandparents did, with Epsom salt and baking soda, as well as whatever skin- and muscle-soothing herbs are appropriate for the occasion: often lavender, calendula, and comfrey, and sometimes additions like oatmeal for extra skin pampering. I also like St. John's wort and arnica flowers when I'm achy, and ginger when I'm feeling a little under the weather and need to warm up. In Ayurvedic tradition, you may see "warmer" herbs and spices like mustard powder included to stimulate skin circulation and rejuvenate tired muscles.

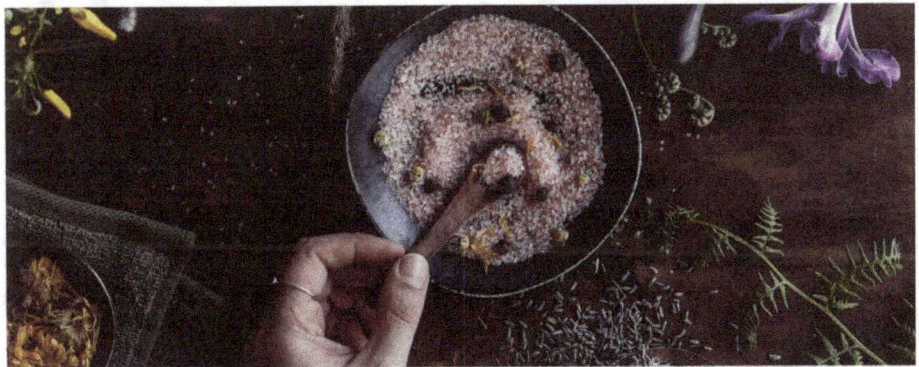

HOW TO MAKE AN HERBAL SITZ BATH IN THE BATHTUB

Ingredients
- 1 to 2 cups Epsom salt per gallon of water, depending on skin sensitivity
- 1/2 to 3/4 cup baking soda per gallon of water
- Up to 1 cup other salts like Himalayan Pink Salt, optional
- Cotton tea net or muslin bag full of organic herbs of choice (approximately 1/2 cup)

Directions
1. Thoroughly scrub your bathtub and rinse it well so there is no soap residue.
2. Adjust water temperature so that it is warm enough to dissolve salt but is not uncomfortably hot.
3. Fill tub with just enough warm water so it will just cover your hips when you sit down. Do not add other oils or soaps.
4. Add Epsom salt, baking soda, optional additional salts, and bag of herbs. Agitate as necessary to dissolve salts and baking powder, and to encourage herbal goodness to seep into the bath. Alternatively, hang herb bag on the drain so the water runs over it as the tub fills.
5. Climb in and soak for 15-20 minutes, making sure to keep the most affected areas of your lower body in the water.
6. Rinse off the salts in fresh water. Gently pat yourself dry.
7. Repeat up to 3-4 times a day, as needed for relief.

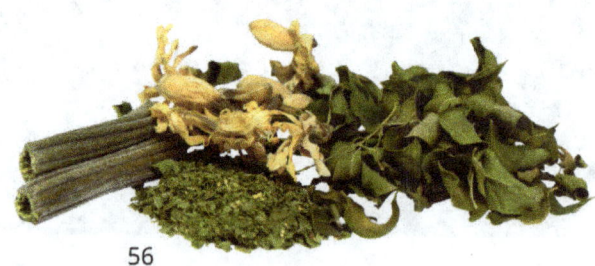

Pro Tips

- If you need to fill the tub a little deeper to reach your lower back, adjust amount of Epsom salt, baking soda, and herbs accordingly for more water.
- You can put herbs directly into your bath water but cleaning them out again can be a pain in your just-soaked backside. A tea net or muslin bag makes cleanup a breeze. If you are using powdered herbs, you'll need to use a muslin bag.
- Remember to rinse the tub after your sitz bath so you don't leave salt behind for the next person.

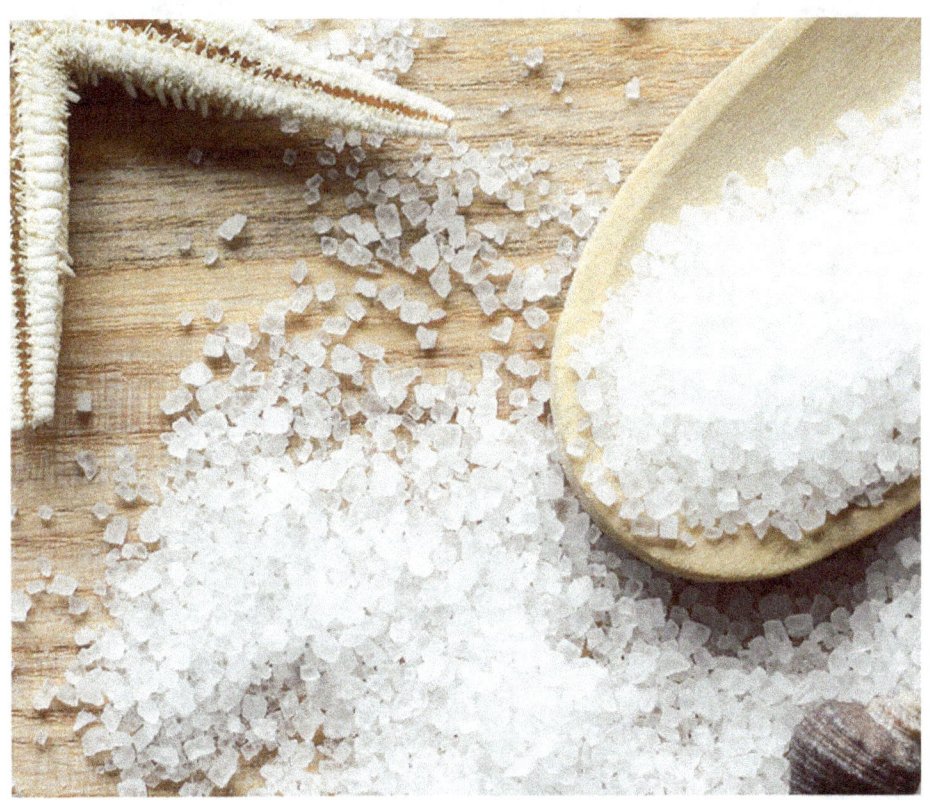

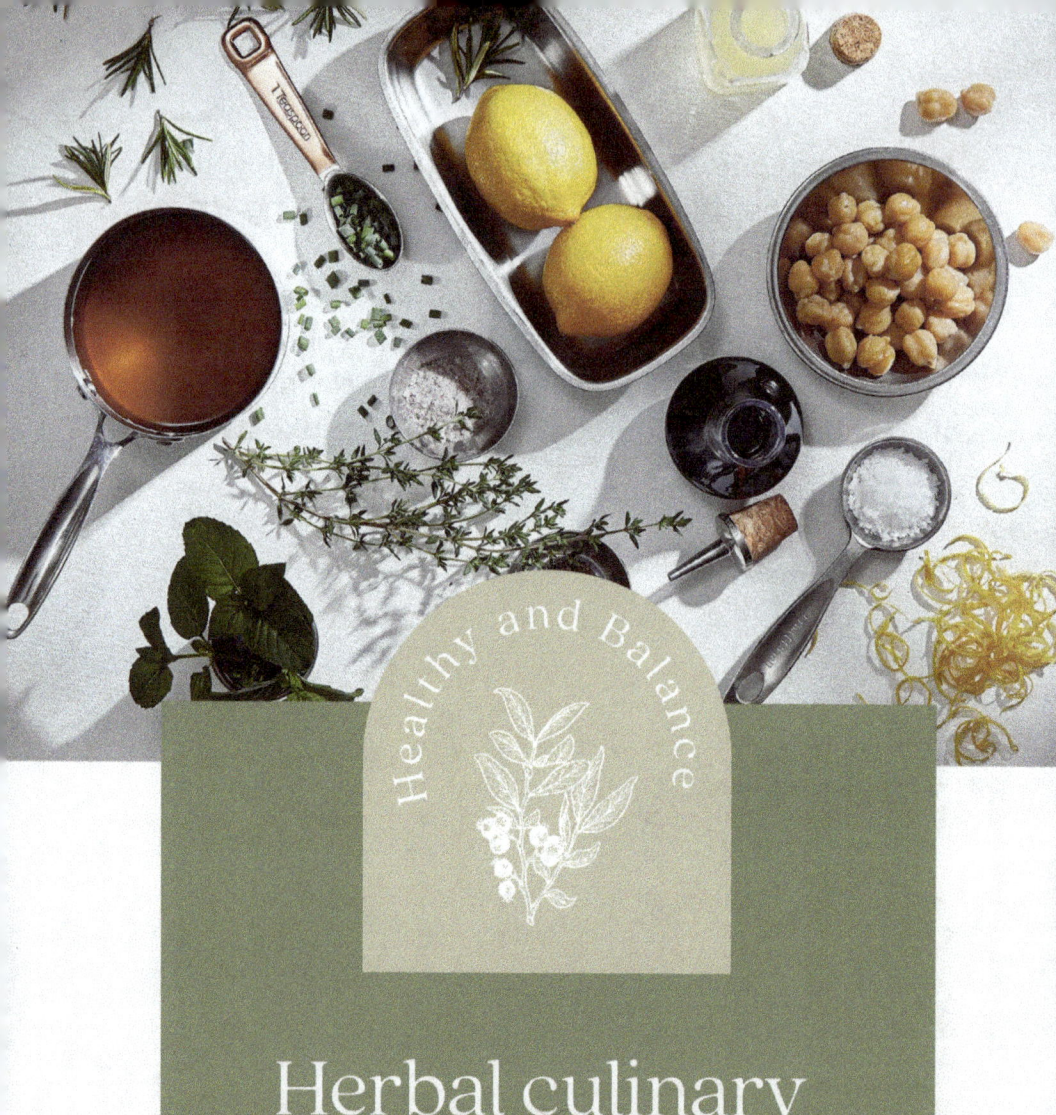

Herbal culinary additions: Sprinkles, Syrups, Bitters & Salt Blends

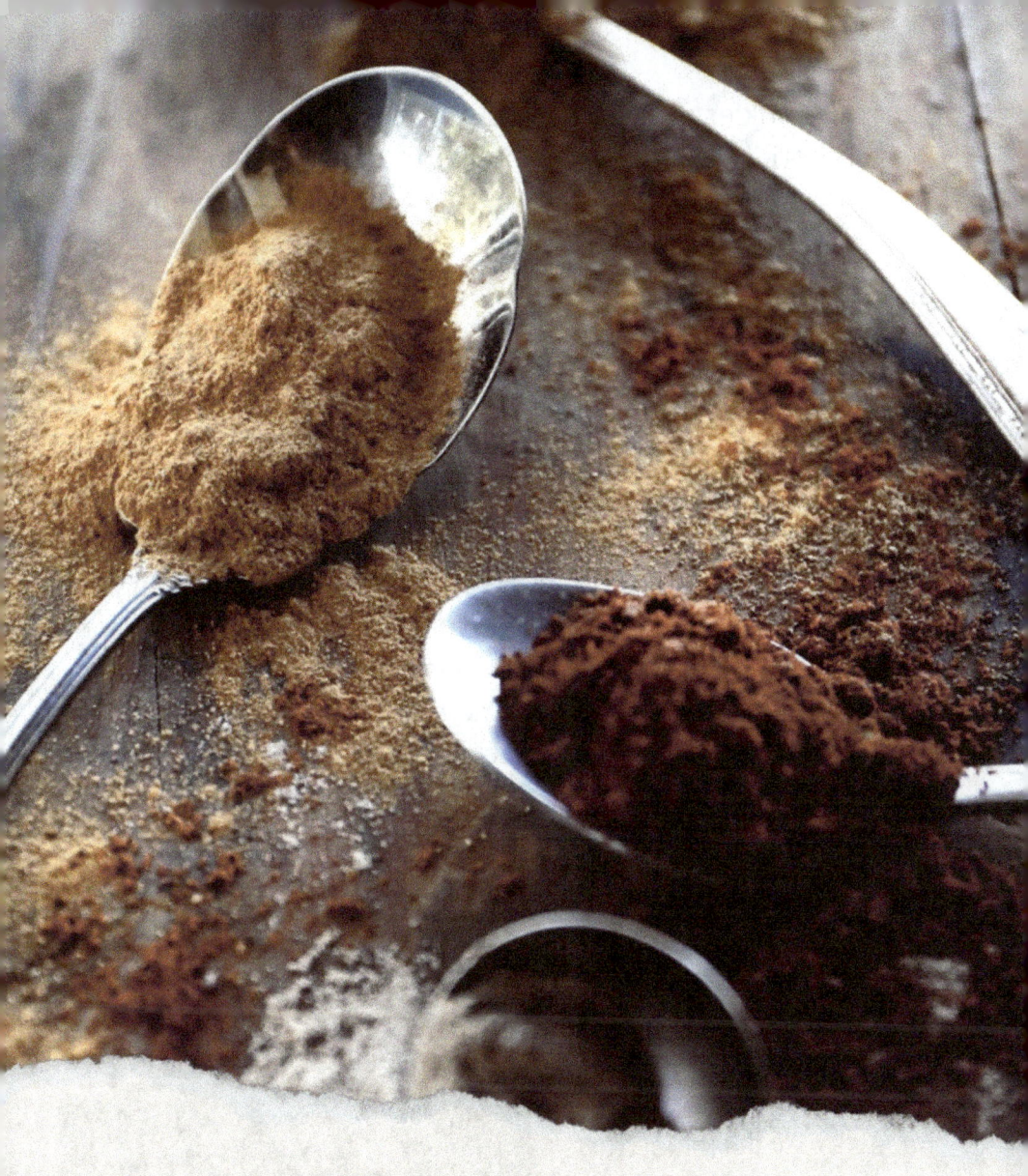

SPRINKLE-ON HERB & SPICE BLENDS FOR FOUR SEASON WELLNESS

Herbal sprinkles are a quick and easy DIY project that will help you fit more healthful herbs into your meals. Instead of having your spices tucked away in the cabinet, keep a few versatile blends on your table, and you'll find that eating herbs at every meal is easy—when they are right in front of you, you can't help but use them! Pretty soon, you'll wonder how you ever got by without such a pleasing array of spices at your fingertips to liven up breakfast, lunch, and dinner.

This post could also be called "Beyond Pepper." No matter where you go, this is the one spice that adorns almost all tables, from homes to cafeterias to fine restaurants: pepper. I used to take for granted the fact that we settled on this one tabletop choice for all of our self-seasoning needs, but dining with my Persian friends (who always keep a shaker full of sumac next to the pepper) got me thinking that it might be nice to have more options. I decided to take my own standard table setup a little further.

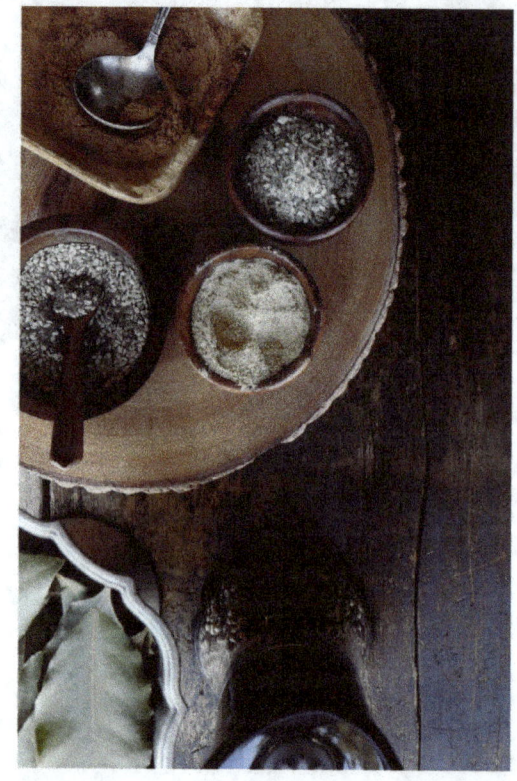

At the beginning of each season, I open up my herb cabinet and mix together half a dozen herbal sprinkle mixtures to use during the coming months. I make sure to have savory sprinkles for salad dressings and marinades, several sweet and aromatic blends that I use lavishly in breakfast foods and treats, and then a couple mixtures that contain specific herbs that I want to work into my diet during that season. We regularly keep about seven shakers of herbs on the table at any given time.

In my house, we started putting herbal sprinkles on a lazy susan for easy seasoning access during meals. It was a hit, and now that lazy susan full of various herbal sprinkles, is a permanent fixture on our kitchen table. Hundreds of people have told me that putting the herbal sprinkles in the dining area has been the single best move for activating interest in herbs among their family members.

The possibilities for herbal sprinkle combinations are endless! But to get you started, here are four popular seasonal herbal sprinkles that I think you will enjoy!

HOW TO MAKE HERBAL SPRINKLES

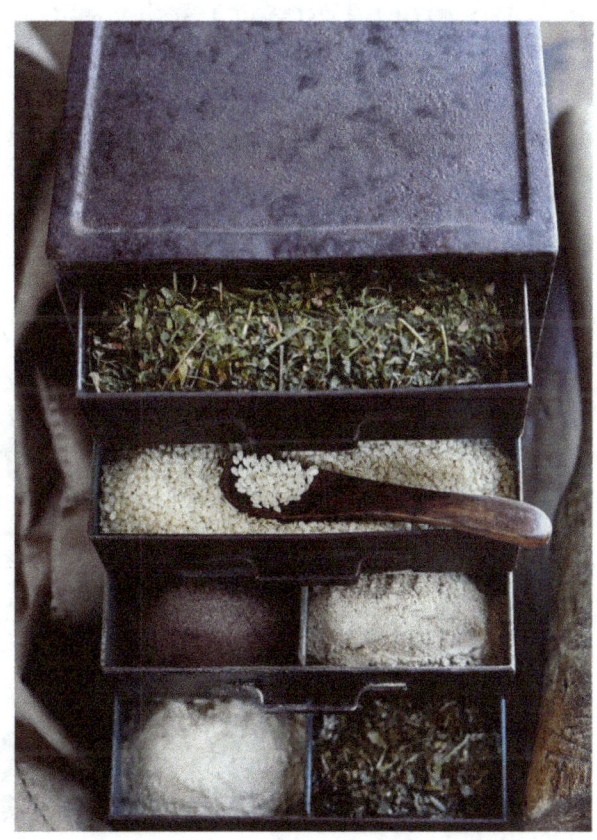

Directions
1. Choose your dried herbs and spices.
2. Mix powdered or hand ground herbs together well in a bowl.
3. Put into a salt shaker.
4. Sprinkle on your food. Easy!

Herb Sprinkle Recipes

LOVE YOUR LIVER SPRINKLE FOR SPRING
As winter's ice begins to thaw and the water starts moving again, the same thing happens in the body. Spring is the time to shed the layers of winter and lighten up a little. Take care of your liver and everything moves with more ease. This liver support mixture is a nice addition to smoothies, salad dressings, and soups.

Ingredients
- 2 Tbsp. whole or ground organic sesame seeds
- 2 Tbsp. ground organic dandelion leaf
- 1 tsp. organic dandelion root powder
- 1 tsp. organic burdock root powder
- 1 tsp. ground organic parsley leaf
- 1 tsp. organic dulse powder

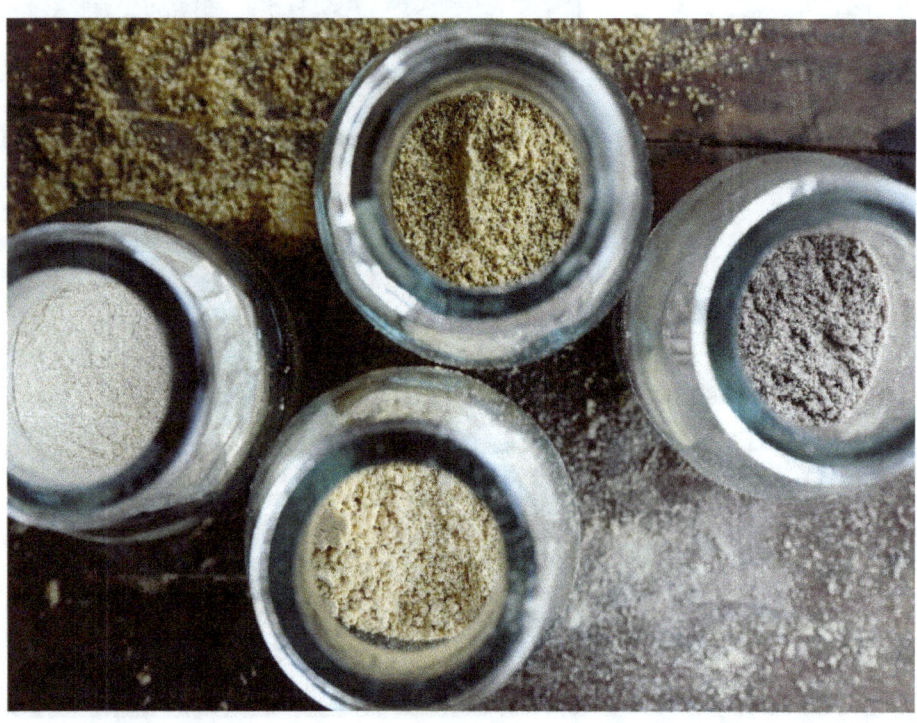

Herb Sprinkle Recipes

LOVE YOUR LIVER SPRINKLE FOR SPRING

As winter's ice begins to thaw and the water starts moving again, the same thing happens in the body. Spring is the time to shed the layers of winter and lighten up a little. Take care of your liver and everything moves with more ease. This liver support mixture is a nice addition to smoothies, salad dressings, and soups.

Ingredients

- 2 Tbsp. whole or ground organic sesame seeds
- 2 Tbsp. ground organic dandelion leaf
- 1 tsp. organic dandelion root powder
- 1 tsp. organic burdock root powder
- 1 tsp. ground organic parsley leaf
- 1 tsp. organic dulse powder

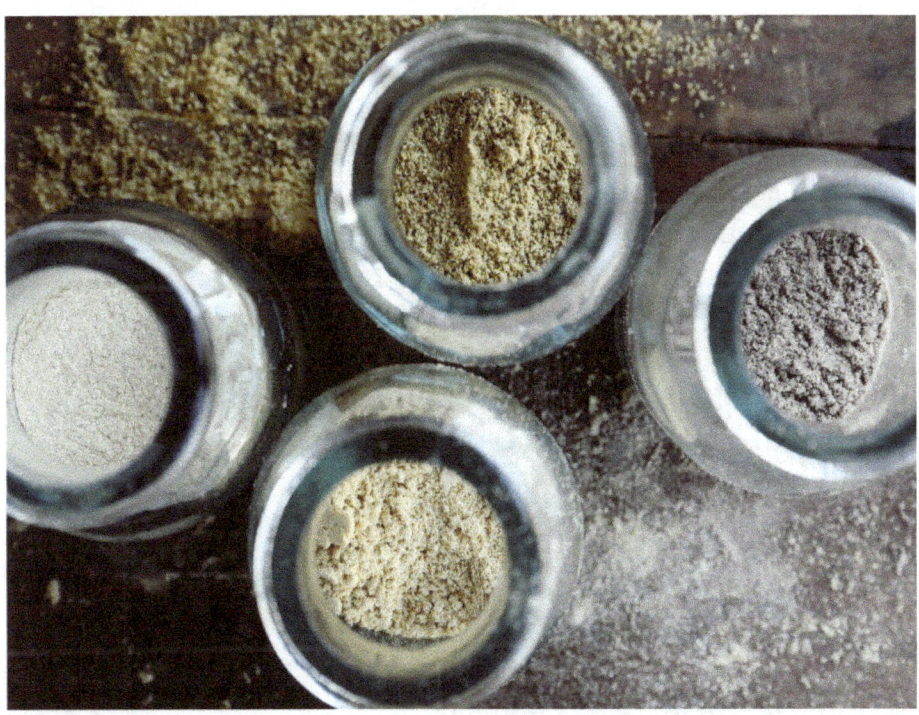

ORANGE SPICE SPRINKLE FOR FALL

This sprinkle can easily be added to drinks and smoothies. That is the great thing about sprinkles—if you have family members that aren't quite as passionate as you are about getting their daily dose of herbs, sprinkles can be slipped in here and there without anyone even knowing! This blend is a good addition to recipes that call for flour: pie crust, muffins, dumplings, cookies, and corn bread. Just add some of the sprinkle to the flour when making the batter. We also sprinkle this on fruit snacks, apple sauce, and desserts.

Ingredients
- 2 Tbsp. organic orange peel powder
- 1 Tbsp. organic fennel powder
- 1/2 tsp. organic ginger powder
- 1/4 tsp. organic cardamom powder

WARMING BREAKFAST SPRINKLE FOR WINTER

As the days grow colder and darker, and we crave more insulating foods, it helps to have a carminative at every meal. This combination of carminative spices helps you digest your food and is an especially useful digestive aid for the heavier fare of winter holiday feasts. This spice blend is good on French toast, muffins, scones, bagels, pancakes, and oatmeal—that's why we call it Breakfast Sprinkle! Since it tends to be a people-pleaser, I like to make up big batches and give it away as gifts.

Ingredients
- 3 Tbsp. organic cinnamon powder
- 1 Tbsp. organic allspice powder
- 1/2 tsp. organic cardamom powder
- 1/2 tsp. organic clove powder

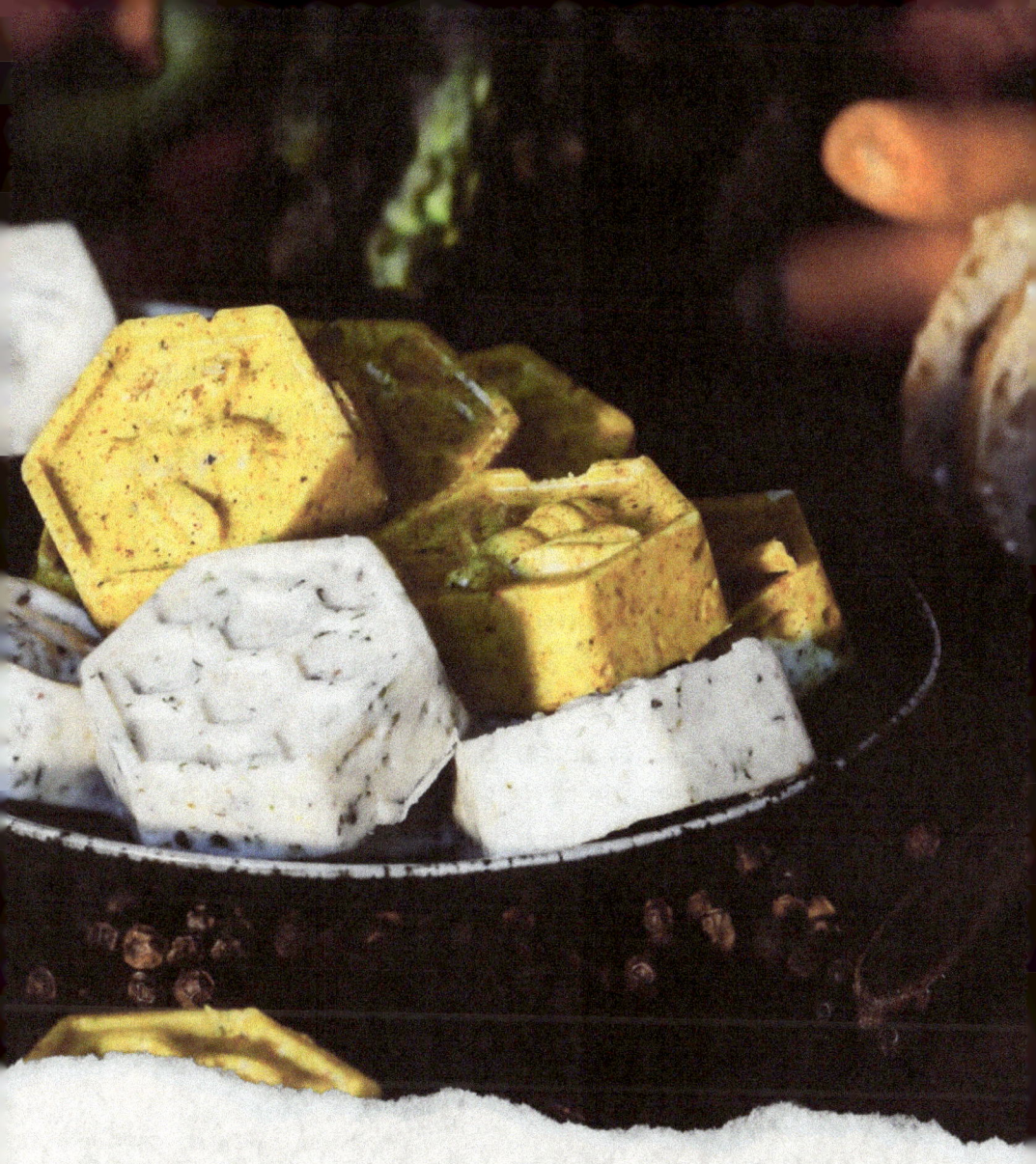

HERBAL COMPOUND
BUTTER RECIPES

Compound butter is believed to be of French origin, though there is no doubt in my mind that herbs have been incorporated into butter and fats long before they were first attributed to fine French cuisine. While butter gets a bad rap for its high fat content, fat is essential for our bodies and like all things in life, it's about moderation! With compound butter, not only are you adding herbs and spices for flavor, but you are also incorporating the beneficial constituents of those plants into your culinary preparations. Am I insinuating that this is a health-food recipe?Not at all. But I do believe that a balanced diet that includes herbs and spices at every turn is important.

In addition to the more functional aspects of cooking, mealtime should be a time of joy—at least that's what my Italian genetics tell me. Even the smallest of gestures, like folding napkins in fancy patterns, lighting candles, or in this case, making homemade herbal butters, can take even the simplest of spreads and make them feel like something really special. This extra little pizazz shows that you put the time and effort into the finer details. You can even take it one step further and make them into shapes that fit the occasion.

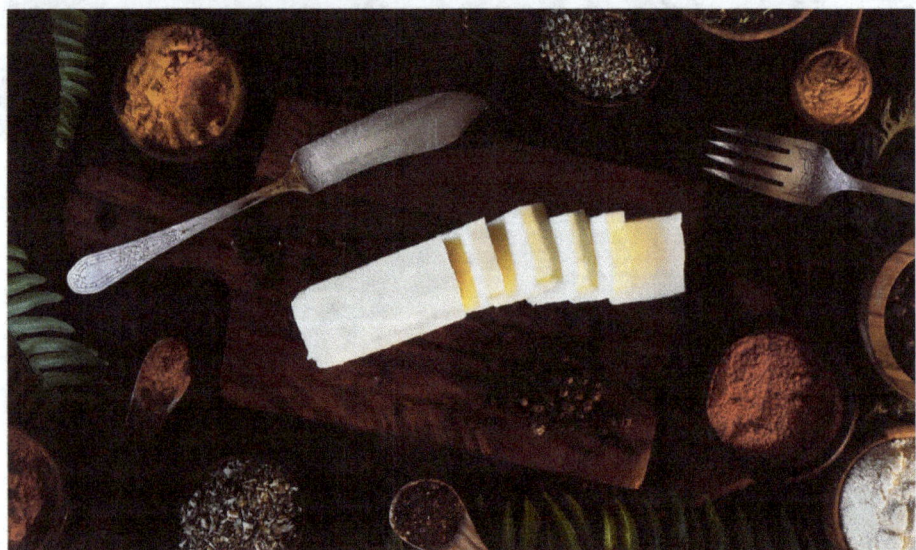

Compound Butter Recipes

ITALIAN HERBAL BUTTER

Makes about 1/2 cup.

Ingredients

- 1/2 cup organic butter or vegan alternative (unsalted)
- 1/4 tsp. organic basil leaf
- 1/4 tsp. organic garlic powder
- 1/4 tsp. organic parsley leaf
- 1/8 tsp. organic oregano leaf
- 1/8-1/4 tsp. salt, to taste (optional)

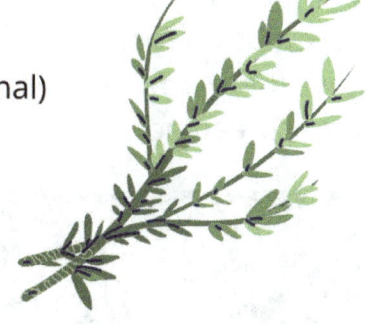

SPICED TURMERIC COMPOUND BUTTER RECIPE

Ingredients

Makes about 1/2 cup.

- 1/2 cup organic butter or vegan alternative (unsalted)
- 1/2 tsp. organic paprika powder
- 1/4 tsp. organic ground peppercorn
- 1/4 tsp. organic turmeric root powder
- 1/8 tsp. organic roasted chili powder
- 1/8-1/4 tsp. smoked salt, to taste (optional)

Directions

Soften butter until it is completely malleable. (Do not melt.)
Add spices and mix together using a fork.
Once completely incorporated, spoon into mold of choice.
Pick up mold and drop it onto counter several times to work
out any air bubbles.
If using within a week, place in refrigerator to harden so they
will pop out of the mold cleanly.
If making ahead of time, place mold in the freezer and once
completely solid, pop out and put in an airtight container for
longer term storage. (Don't forget to label!)
Pro tip: If using them on the dinner table, remember to
remove them from the fridge or freezer early enough to be
soft for spreading.

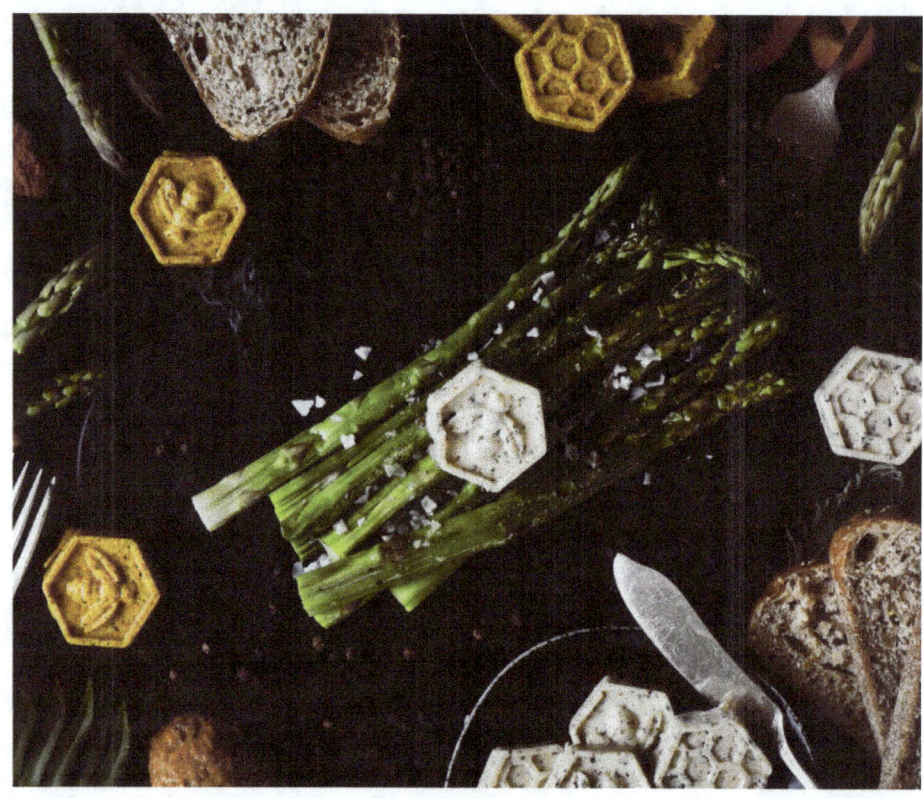

How to Use Compound Butters

You can use compound butter any way you would use regular butter, but here are some of my favorites!

- Spread on bread or toast
- As a cooking fat for morning eggs
- Sautee base for vegetables
- As a flavoring and cooking fat for fish, meat, or protein of choice
- Grilled cheese
- Macaroni and cheese
- Mashed potatoes
- Baked potatoes
- Corn on the cob

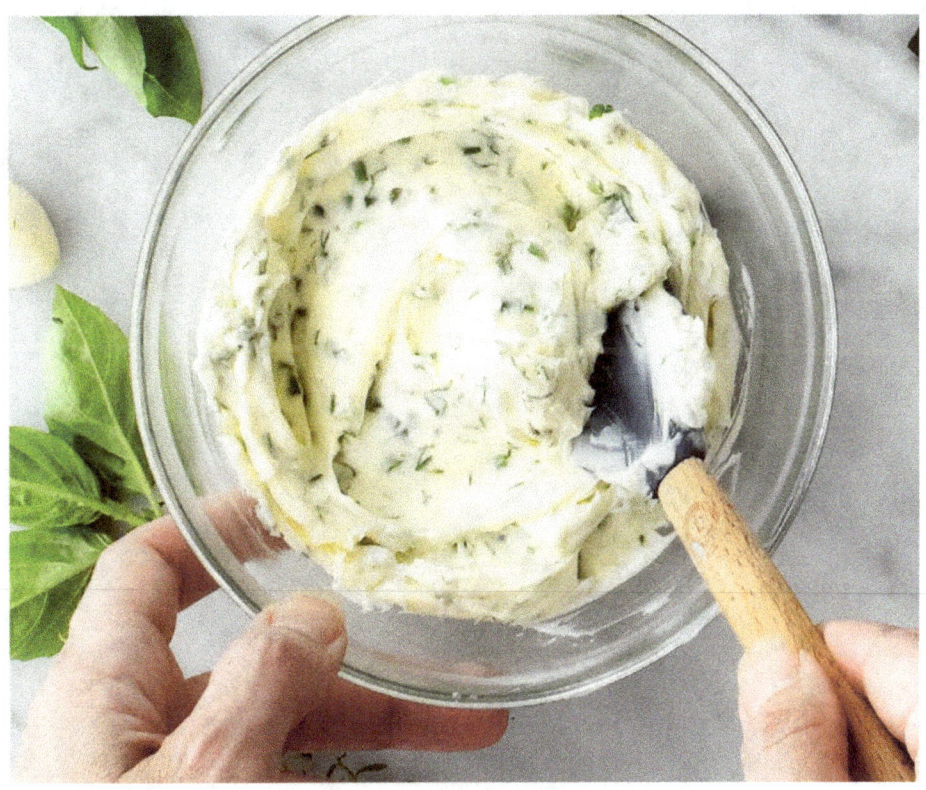

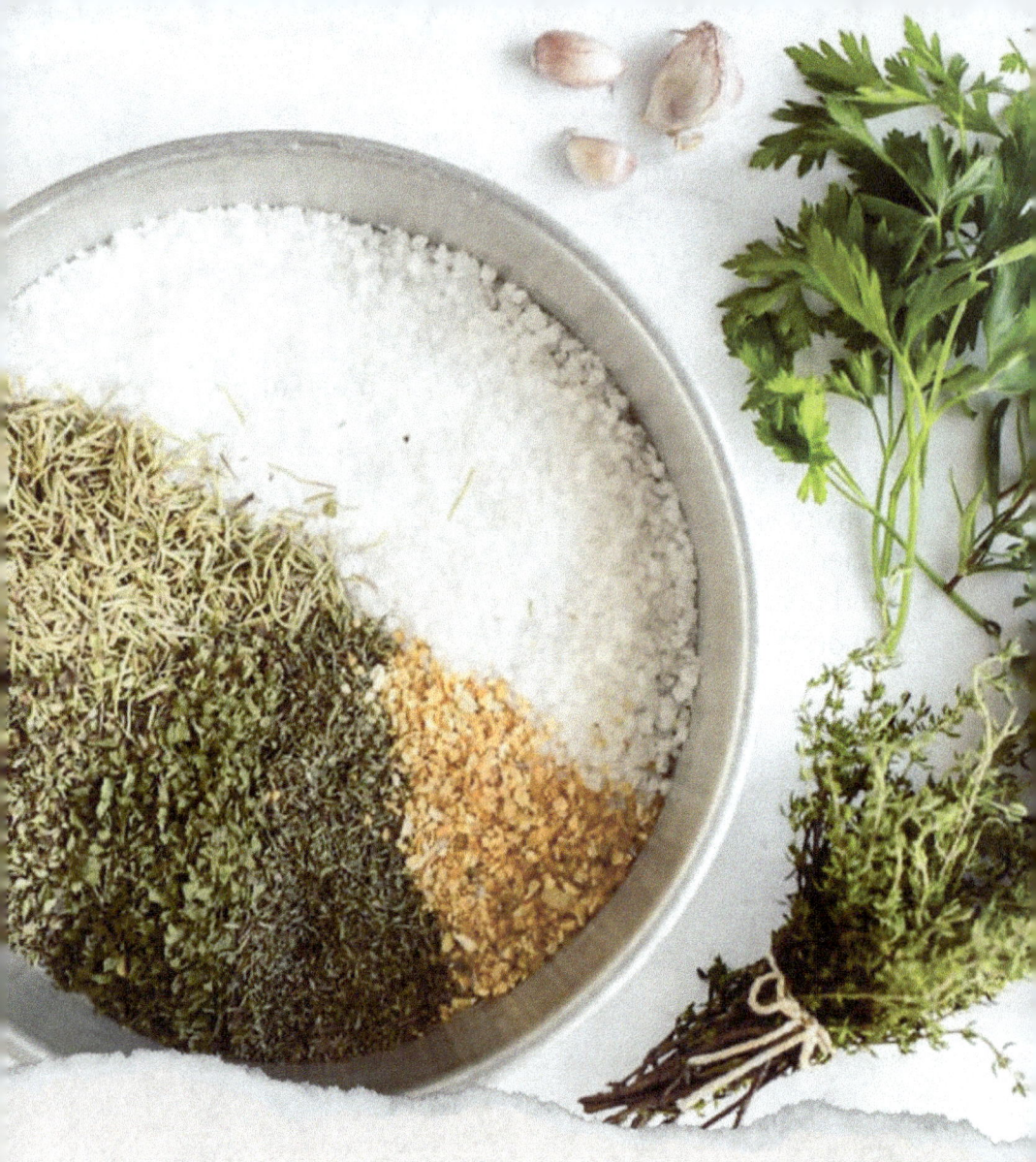

HOW TO MAKE HERBAL SALT BLENDS

It is mighty cliché to start a health and wellness blog with a Hippocrates quote, but I am willing to sacrifice originality for truth. The old adage "Let food be thy medicine and medicine be thy food" is still worthy of repeating some 2,400 years after it was first uttered and despite centuries of medical and health advances, it is still relevant today. In this modern age, especially in America, many of us are living with nutritional deficiencies and are at a higher risk of experiencing food-related illnesses.

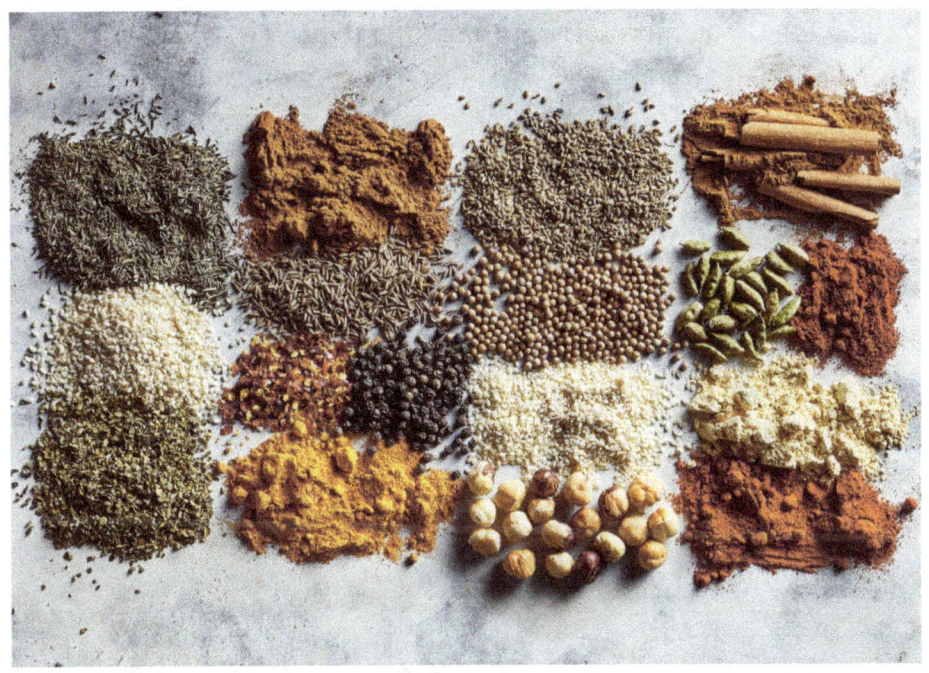

Jump to Recipe

While the list of reasons contributing to this growing problem is long and complex, I like to remain solution-oriented and do what I can to prevent, or at least minimize my risks. I'm not perfect when it comes to my diet, but I can easily commit to simple changes that add more nutrient-dense plants and health-supporting mushrooms. After all, it is the day in and day out wellness routines that really have lasting effects.

This is why I started adding health-promoting ingredients to a staple I use often—salt. You might now be asking why I am recommending the use of salt in a blog on health. Salt, in and of itself, is essential for the human diet, and as with most things in life, it's all about moderation!

According to the Center for Disease Control, the average American consumes 30% more than the recommended salt intake. Replacing table salt with herbal salt results in consuming less of it while increasing the nutritional value of your meals. You'll notice in the recipes below that the salt-to-herb ratio is roughly 30%. This of course can be tailored to your taste, but I found the flavor to be in perfect balance and the ratio seemed to be in divine proportion.

I hope that these recipes serve as a starting point for you to get comfortable with the idea of homemade salt blends so that you can start customizing them based on your needs.

Wishing you many healthy meals surrounded by those you love.

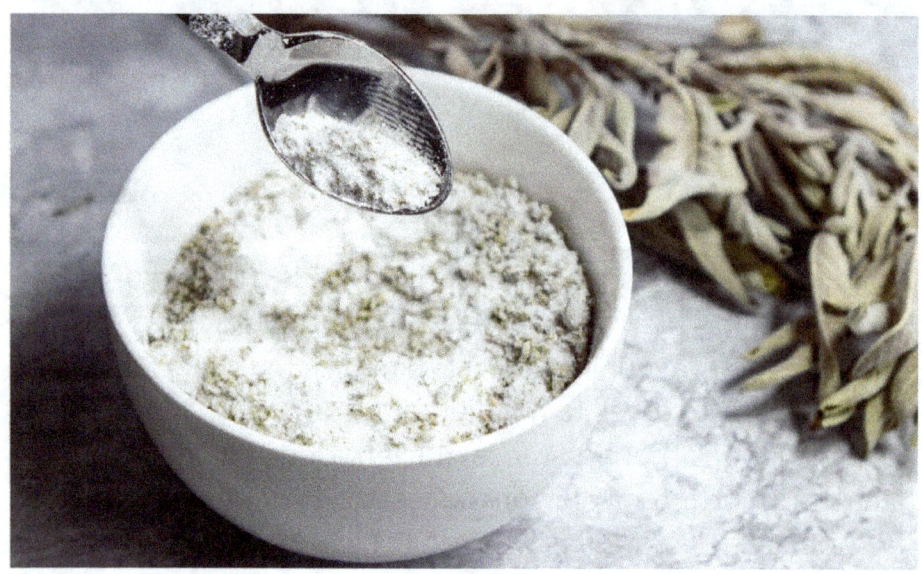

Nutrient-Packed Green Salt Recipe

- 2 tsp. fine sea salt
- 1 tsp. organic nettle leaf powder
- 1 tsp. organic alfalfa powder
- 1 tsp. organic spinach leaf powder
- 1 tsp. organic kale powder
- 1 1/2 tsp. organic spirulina powder

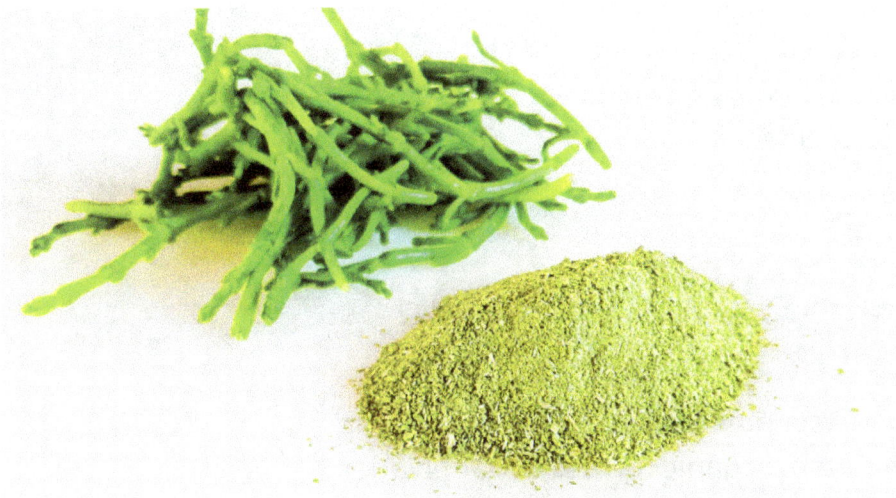

Adaptogenic Mushroom Salt Recipe

- 2 tsp. fine sea salt
- 1 tsp. organic shiitake mushroom powder
- 1 tsp. organic cordyceps powder
- 1 tsp. organic chaga mushroom powder
- 1 tsp. astragalus root powder

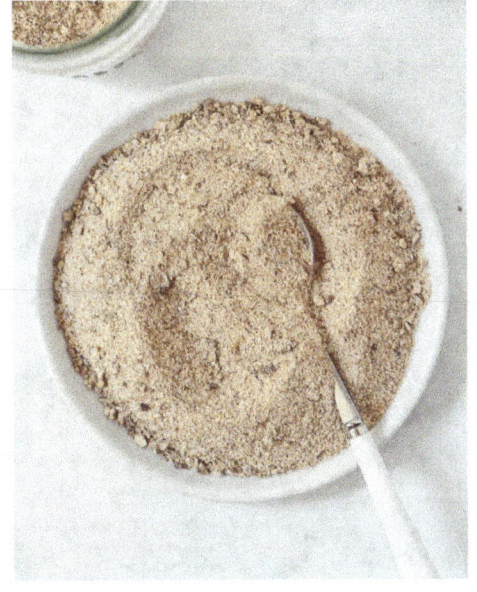

Antioxidant Red Salt Recipe

- 2 tsp. red alaea salt
- 1 tsp. organic red roasted chili powder
- 1 tsp. organic paprika powder
- 1 tsp. organic beet root powder
- 1 tsp. organic garlic powder

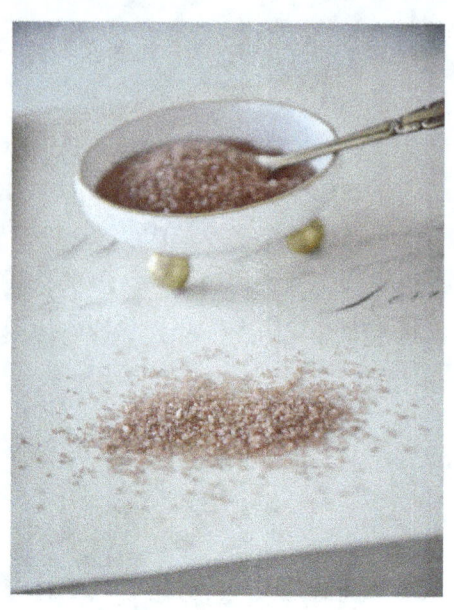

Joint-Supporting Turmeric Recipe (Low-Salt)

- 1 tsp. pink Himalayan salt
- 2 tsp. organic turmeric root powder
- 1 tsp. organic black pepper
- 1 tsp. organic ginger root powder

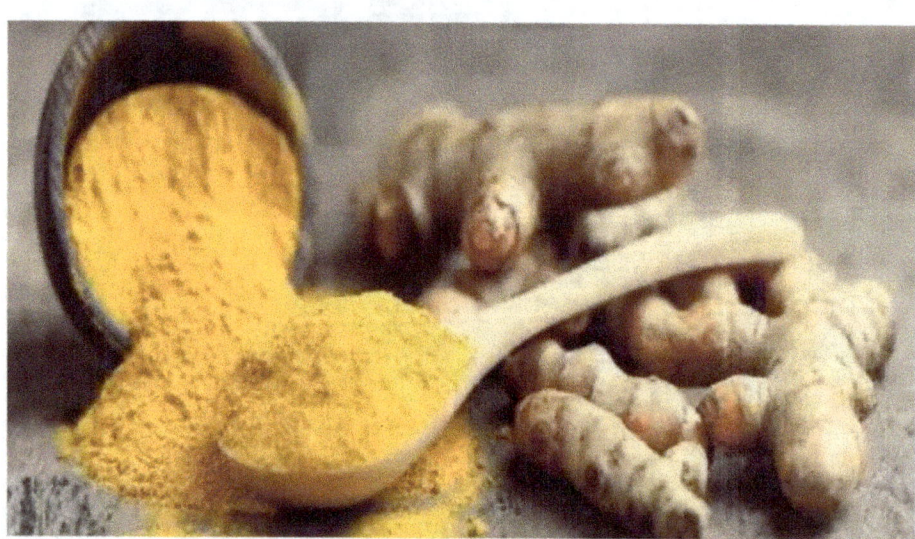

Directions

- Thoroughly mix ingredients in a bowl and store in an airtight spice bottle.
- Label with ingredients and date to ensure optimal freshness.

To use: Add blends to your cooking in place of straight salt. They can also replace your table salt.

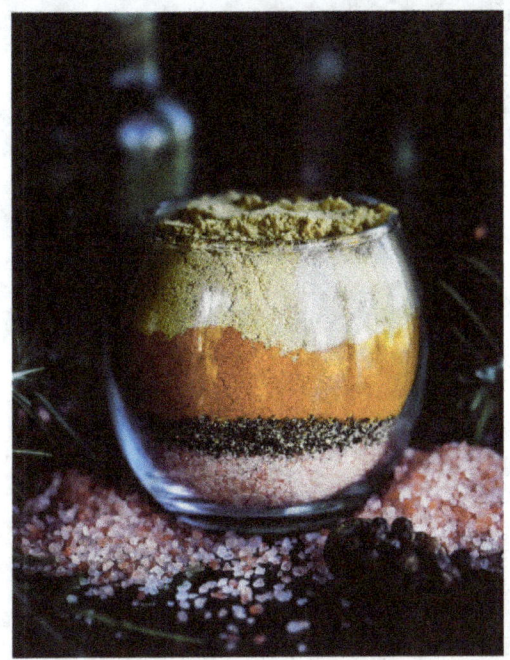

Pro Tips

- If ingredients aren't powdered to the same size grind, I recommend blending them all together either in a spice grinder or with a mortar and pestle. This will ensure a more even mixture when adding to food.
- Having several blends made up in advance offers a wider variety of flavors to meld with different dishes.
- It's a good idea to switch up your herbs so that your body can benefit from the varying vitamins and minerals.
- You can substitute some of the salt for seaweed powder to boost the nutritional benefit. However, keep in mind that seaweed contains naturally occurring iodine. While also necessary for optimal health, the National Institute of Health recommends that most adults not exceed 150 micrograms of iodine per day so adding seaweed powder to all of your meals may not be ideal.
- When adding new herbal ingredients to your health regimen, we recommend doing research and consulting with a healthcare practitioner to ensure that the new ingredients will complement your individual needs.

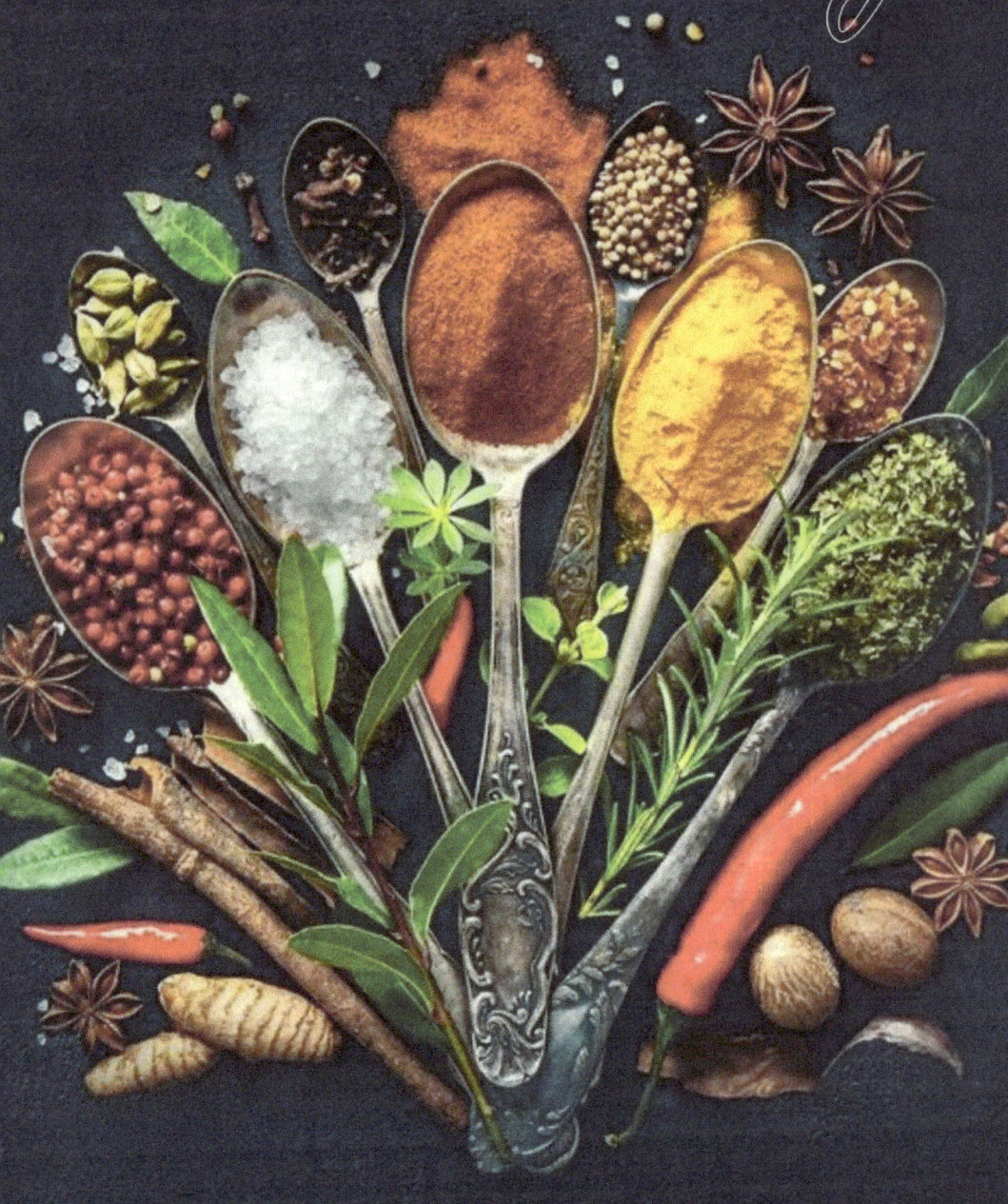

Thanks for reading